MEDIEVAL MEDICUS

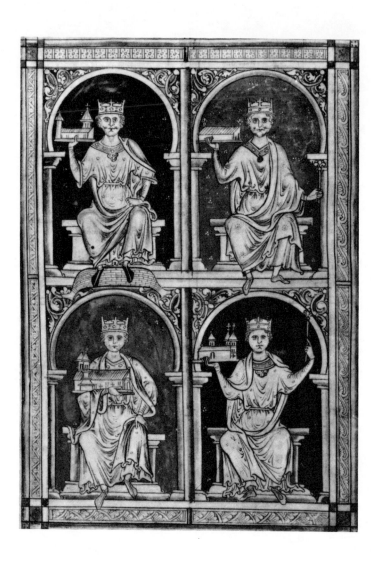

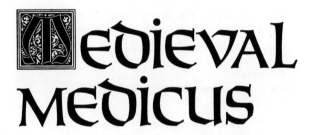

MEDIEVAL MEDICUS

A SOCIAL HISTORY
OF ANGLO-NORMAN
MEDICINE

by Edward J. Kealey

THE JOHNS HOPKINS UNIVERSITY PRESS : BALTIMORE AND LONDON

This book has been brought to publication with the generous assistance of the Andrew F. Mellon Foundation.

The Johns Hopkins University Press, Baltimore, Maryland 21218
The Johns Hopkins Press Ltd., London

Library of Congress Cataloging in Publication Data
Kealey, Edward J.
  Medieval medicus.
  Bibliography: p. 163
  Includes index.
  1. Medicine, Medieval — England. 2. Physicians — England —
Biography. 3. Hospitals, Medieval — England. 4. England — Social
conditions — Medieval period, 1066–1485. I. Title. [DNLM:
1. History of medicine, Medieval — England. 2. Physicians —
England — Biography. WZ70 FE5 K24m]
R141.K4   362.1'0942   80-21870
ISBN 0-8018-2533-4

The thirteenth-century chronicler Matthew Paris envisioned the Anglo-Norman kings — William I, William II, Henry I, and Stephen — as pictured on the frontispiece. Each ruler holds aloft a model of one of his principal ecclesiastical charities. By permission of the British Library, Ms. Royal 14 C VII, fo. 158.

The characters introducing each chapter are physicians and cautery men from a collection of medical and astrological treatises made in Durham between 1100 and 1128. For other drawings from the same manuscript, see illustration on p. 48. By permission of the Dean and Chapter of Durham Cathedral, Ms. Hunter 100, fos. 119v–20.

To
JACK AND HELEN,
BOB,
DON AND MARGARET

CONTENTS

ILLUSTRATIONS

PREFACE

Many stimulating writers have already surveyed broad vistas of medieval social and medical history, but a tighter focus, the health services truly available within a single lifespan, can be equally instructive. The years 1100–54 not only constitute such a realistic interval, but in England they also encompass an exciting, constructive moment in social progress.

My study of that age is divided into two parts. Narrative chapters examine the unprecedented Anglo-Norman demand for better medical care, the diverse careers of identifiable physicians, and the public support of nursing facilities. Appendixes document the occurrences of each practitioner and list the establishment of all local hospitals. The evidence for this period is buried amidst the charters and chronicles that so uniquely preserve Britain's heritage. Digging out the details, bit by bit, simulates some of the pleasures of archaeological excavation and detective investigation. Initial results may appear fragmentary, but eventually patterns can emerge to recreate a mosaic of human experience.

Discovering these fascinating people, both the rascals and the reformers, has been fun and I am genuinely indebted to many individuals for insight and assistance. I owe most to scholars whose publication of original records and historical syntheses enabled me to undertake this exploration. I trust I compliment them by freely incorporating their conclusions into my own presentation. In particular, I am grateful to Professor Christopher R. Cheney of Corpus Christi College, Cambridge University, for special help generously volunteered. The College of the Holy Cross, Worcester, Massachusetts, awarded a faculty fellowship to complete this study, and Saint Edmund's

House, Cambridge University, graciously hosted my overseas research. Talented individuals at the Johns Hopkins University Press, especially Susan Bishop, Anders Richter, and Miriam Tillman, offered valuable creative advice.

Twelfth-century people were continually urged to heed the advice of three sages — Doctor Diet, Doctor Quiet, and Doctor Merryman. May the last physician, at least, guide us all.

MEDIEVAL MEDICUS

I. MIRACLES, MARVELS, AND MONARCHS

Expanded health care is one of the unheralded glories of twelfth-century England. In fact, the country may have enjoyed better access to medical service between 1100 and 1154 than at any other time until the twentieth century. This authentic achievement went unacclaimed partly because medieval observers exaggerated their own dependence on classical standards and partly because modern analysts equated medical progress exclusively with scientific expertise or surgical technique. A fresh look at the records, however, reveals a far greater measure of Anglo-Norman success.

Contributing to this accomplishment were a large, multitalented medical fraternity, a compassionate diocesan and monastic clergy, and a public-spirited royal entourage. Hundreds of other English men and women merit equal praise for their generous support of almshouses, nursing homes, and voluntary hospitals. This story is therefore about many people—princes, peasants, bishops, barons, monks, merchants, wives, and widows. As physician, patient, or patron each played a role, and sometimes their important but unrecognized sacrifices still echo in empty halls.

Offering medical assistance was often a frustrating and exhausting effort. The sick, the injured, and the dying, the poor, the old, and the disoriented, are difficult to help in the best of times, but how were they to be housed and comforted in an age of limited resources? Charitable responses always vary

1

with knowledge, facilities, and skill, but they are most affected by the values that different cultures place upon human life.

Fortunately, medieval European society was firmly grounded in one strong religious faith, which emphasized the primacy of individual persons and eagerly provided explanations for the ultimate goals of existence. By the twelfth century, innovative leaders were also wrestling with the challenges of immediate public welfare and struggling to embody their high ideals in lasting community services.

The experiments in England reflect the quest of all Christendom and yet possess unique local features. Some of the best ideas bore great fruits that endure to this day. Other opportunities never matured at all, as false leads, changed directions, and civil strife withered their prospects with untimely speed.

During the decades after William the Conqueror's victory in 1066, England and Normandy developed similar institutions and usually shared the same ruler. A strong argument can therefore be made for considering the two lands a united realm. About ten thousand Normans migrated to Britain, but they retained ancestral rights at home and many, including several doctors, often revisited the duchy. Others came too, including large numbers of Flemings and Bretons and a trickle of Germans and Italians. Nevertheless, in many fields native Saxon practices continued to outweigh the Norman genius for administration and the continental flair for theoretical scholarship. So it was in medicine; although most known physicians had Norman names, medical manuscripts usually had Saxon associations. Within a generation, however, the separate traditions were intermingling and producing their own novel effects, including an awakened interest in realistic observation. Such mixed parentage and unusual progeny partially justify isolating consideration of health services to the island kingdom alone.

Limiting analysis to a single brief period can also be revealing. Rather than summarize the disjointed experience of several centuries, this focus concentrates on what care was truly offered to real patients. The combined reigns of Kings Henry I and Stephen, 1100–54, constitute such a viable unit. These are also years that produced beneficial social change. Documents and other evidence are unusually complete, as such things go, and can highlight the period from angles as varied as art, archaeology, biography, ecclesiology, and economics.

Above all, these fifty-four years span an era when something genuinely significant was happening in English public health. Consider just two sets of statistics:

Period	400–1066	1066–1100	1100–1154
Identifiable physicians	8	11	90
Known hospitals	7	21	113

Even granting the low base and the uneven survival of sources, the accelerating rate of Anglo-Norman progress was truly remarkable.[1] Although it is easier to quantify such results than to articulate their motives, the figures do indicate that a new spirit was alive in the country. Before examining its effect on the careers of Anglo-Norman practitioners, however, something should be said about the environment in which they worked—that is, about the general health of the English people, the scientific books they read and wrote, and the specific interests that inspired courtiers and clergymen to become involved in health care.

Individuals are certainly prey for countless maladies, and famine particularly cursed the Saxons, especially in the "hungry forties" of Edward the Confessor's reign; otherwise, they were a fairly lucky people.[2] When a nationwide epidemic finally did strike, King William hurriedly left England for Normandy. His physicians recommended a regimen of severe dieting, but then King Philip I of France ridiculed his large-chested, overweight rival, laughing that William kept to his bed like a woman in childbirth. In humiliation the weakened Conqueror angrily rose up, attacked a rebellious town, and fatally ruptured his own stomach in the assault. Distinguished representatives of the medical professions of England and Normandy hastened to his aid, but they could only check his urine and, perhaps finding therein the blood of internal injuries, helplessly watch him expire.[3]

Like their father, the sons of the Conqueror did not fare well in death. William Rufus fell sick in 1093 and, thinking he was about to die, penitently chose saintly Anselm of Bec for the long-vacant archbishopric of Canterbury. William recovered, but on the first of August, 1100, this second Norman king supposedly had a nightmare that he was being bled by a surgeon and that the stream of his blood gushed to heaven, clouding the skies. The following day, while hunting in the New Forest, an arrow pierced his throat, and this gifted but controversial monarch died without a word. His brother Richard had perished in the same area some time before. Decades later, another brother, Robert Curthose, once duke of Normandy but for twenty-one years prisoner of yet another brother, reportedly foresaw his only heir's death in battle and languished on for six more lonely years of confinement.

The Conqueror's fourth son, Henry, the jailer of his brother Robert, enjoyed a long reign of varied accomplishment, but his first wife passed away after eighteen years of marriage and his one legitimate son was shipwrecked and drowned while returning from his wedding on the Continent. In 1135, against the advice of his physicians, Henry feasted on eels, took sick, and died. His troubled successor, Stephen, grandson of the Conqueror, ruled for nineteen trying years and died quietly in 1154, conscious of his own failures and his inability to pass the throne to his one surviving son.

Although the deaths of these princes were thus as unpredictable and occasionally as ignoble as those of their least renowned subjects, Anglo-Norman rulers usually had considerable regard for contemporary medical opinion. Perhaps they were motivated by necessity as well as interest.

Despite its achievements, King Henry's reign was not very salubrious. The weather was hard and agricultural yields were low in 1103, 1105, 1110–11, 1116–18, and there was a terrible famine in 1124–25. There were also cattle plagues in 1103, 1111–12, 1115, 1125, and 1131. Worst of all, leprosy, or what was misdiagnosed as leprosy, unaccountably increased.[4] For centuries this disease had attacked very few Britons, but at about the time of the Norman Conquest it began to scourge mounting numbers of the population. It bedeviled Britain and all the West for almost three centuries before curiously fading back to relative quiescence.

Open to question, however, is whether conditions were actually deteriorating or whether twelfth-century people were analyzing their own experience more acutely. Some chronicle entries reporting major disasters surely indicate countrywide tragedy, but others probably generalize from local mishaps. Certainly the national population steadily rose, grandiose construction projects moved ahead swiftly, and the kingdom basked in the blessings of peace. However, the need for improved health care had become obvious to many people.

Fortunately, several modern scholars have recently offered valuable surveys of the full range of English medieval medicine.[5] From them it is clear that late Anglo-Saxon practice and its Anglo-Norman descendant were creative amalgams of valid empirical technique, ancient classical precedent, superstitious ritual incantation, and persuasive psychosomatic faith healing. As in every age, the gamut ran from ludicrous chicanery through clinical observation to tested remedy. Despite some emphasis on folklore and magic, many of the procedures were quite advanced for the time. In fact, the popular interpretation that Europeans at the great medical school of Salerno possessed knowledge superior to that of the Saxons is no longer tenable. Some books that supposedly once signaled a more rational Salernitan approach to treatment in the eleventh century were actually used in England two hundred years earlier.[6] On the other hand, revolting herbal concoctions can occasionally be traced beyond the English gullability that reproduced them to the ancient pseudo-science that originated them.

More commonly, diagnosis was based upon a serious consideration of pain, fever, pulse, and urine. Following the revered concepts of Hippocrates and Galen, bodily disease was usually attributed to an imbalance in one of the four traditional humors: blood, phlegm, yellow bile and black bile. Such excess supposedly colored one's urine and could thereby be detected. A correct balance was called a *tempermantum*. Bloodletting, or phlebotomy, was a regular therapeutic practice in monastic infirmaries as well as among secular clerks and the laity. No harm resulted and it probably constituted a type of preventive medicine by encouraging periodic rest.[7] The Anglo-Normans seemed more interested in proper diet than were the Saxons, but few nutritional specifics were given.

Although arthritis and rheumatism were common disabilities, herbals and leechbooks prescribed more remedies for conditions affecting the eyes than for any other single complaint. Ocular studies had a very long history in England. In Caesar's time there was a famous Celtic eye surgeon in Britain, a man named Ariovist, perhaps the first physician identifiable by name on the island. Eye disease was also disproportionately evident during the ensuing Roman occupation. Numerous prescriptions by opticians have survived, and one British oculist, named Stolus, even had his eye salve mentioned by Galen. Perhaps the prevalence of such disease was caused by a vitamin deficiency, perhaps even by the omnipresent smoke of candle and hearth. Twelfth-century manuscript illustrations suggest that cataract operations were frequently performed, but they were not described in the accompanying texts. Since a number of prominent men were nicknamed "monoculus," it is clear that not all conditions were curable.[8]

Critical observation of different phenomena was, however, more evident in Anglo-Norman Britain than it had been for centuries. The desire for accurate records, so evident in Domesday Book, had great spillover effects. Late Romanesque sculpture, high relief wax seals, and bright manuscript miniatures paraded realistic animal and vegetable forms, and the simultaneous passion for historical research nurtured a love of careful investigation. To their credit, rather than slavishly copy all classical authorities verbatim, some early English scribes annotated or even altered texts to conform to their own experience.[9]

Even though parchment was expensive and all treatises were laboriously transcribed by hand, the book trade flourished in the twelfth century as never before. Theological and liturgical works constituted the bulk of all manuscripts, but hagiography and history also held major portions. Behind them came deeds, accounts, and surveys. Thereafter writers of natural science claimed an increasing share of the market. For this commerce, classical medical texts were avidly reproduced, expanded, revised, illustrated, purchased, and circulated. After the Conquest notable little libraries were acquired by many religious houses, especially Abingdon, Bury, Canterbury, Dover, Durham, and York. Physicians like Clarembald of Exeter, Herbert of Durham, and Ralph of Lincoln even built up personal collections. Indeed, more medical books survive in England from 1100 to 1200 than for the previous six centuries combined. The Anglo-Norman years witnessed a decline in the production of English-language texts, but the output of Latin copies doubled.[10]

Medical treatiese often formed sections of larger scientific compendia. One typical encyclopedic collection of sixty items was made about 1110 for

Thorney Abbey in Cambridgeshire, probably by a Saxon monk. It contains studies on bloodletting (the best time was from April to July on a day not divisible by five), the four humors, weights and measures, abacus calculation, prognostication, and runic letters. Also included were a set of astronomical tables, a list of etymologies and rules of grammar, a glossary of herbs, a Saxon charm against nosebleed, a list of diseases and their remedies, and some recipes for plasters and syrupy electuaries. There were maps of the world with Jerusalem at the center, and of the climactic zones; a diagram, based upon Bede, of the movement of the planets; and a computation that 6,309 years had elapsed between the fall of Adam and A.D. 1100. There were schematic drawings of the various branches of learning, of the degrees of consanguinity which might prevent intermarriage, and of the so-called physical and physiological fours.

The last diagram was copied from a work of Byrhtferth of Ramsay (d. 1011) and acknowledged his authorship. The attractive scheme attempted to demonstrate the relationships and parallels between the four elements, humors, parts of the body (head, chest, belly, and bladder), seasons of the year, ages of man, points of the compass, and signs of the zodiac (twelve signs in four groups). A simpler outline of the same quaternary concepts, probably based upon Isidore of Seville (d. 636), was also included in this corpus. The obsession with numerical symmetry even required fevers to be divided into four great types. Much of the large, miscellaneous collection is traceable directly to Bede and ultimately to classical authorities such as Hippocrates and Galen, but certain elements also paralleled current studies at Salerno, especially the strong emphasis on theoretical rather than experiential knowledge. In sum, the contents of this book indicate what was being read about science and suggest the range of information on subjects other than theology, literature, and history that a great monastery thought it ought to possess.[11]

Critical observation, however, was becoming increasingly evident in the herbals. These descriptive catalogs listed the botanical and therapeutic properties of hundreds of plants and were essential to any physician's pharmacology. Such compilations had an ancient history and were well known to the Saxons, but in the twelfth century they acquired more systematic organization and accurate colored illustrations. For example, the monastic scriptorium at Bury Saint Edmunds in Suffolk, which was evidently begun under the physician-abbot, Baldwin, produced splendid books in many fields. A medical text made there before 1120 contained an elegant copy of the fifth-century Latin herbal of Apuleius Barbarus, a series of extracts from another herbal by the Greek Dioscorides with somewhat cruder drawings, a small collection of medical recipes, a fragment of a law book, and an illustrated copy of the treatise ascribed to Sextus Placitus dealing with remedies derivable from animals.[12]

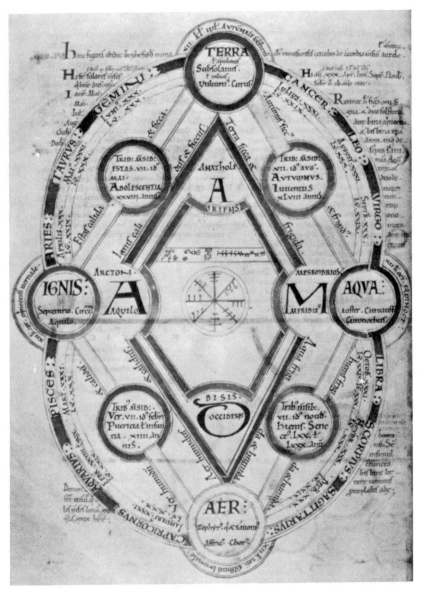

THE PHYSICAL AND PHYSIOLOGICAL FOURS

Diagrams of the organization of nature were common features in medieval encyclopedias. Several were modeled on a scheme developed by Byrhtferth of Ramsey about 1101, which harmonized the four seasons, ages of man, elements, temperaments, compass directions, and signs of the zodiac. This particular version was made for Thorney Abbey either in its own scriptorium or at nearby Ramsey between 1080 and 1110. By permission of the President and Fellows of Saint John's College, Oxford, Ms. 17, fo. 7v.

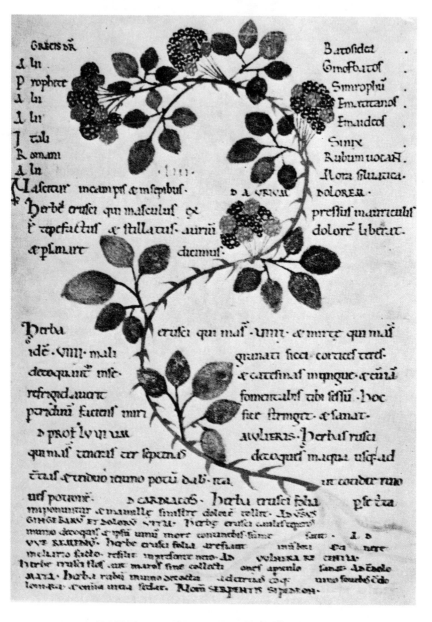

NATURALISM IN SCIENTIFIC ART

Herbals were major components of most physicians' libraries, but the copy executed at Bury
Saint Edmunds Abbey about 1100 is clearly exceptional; it is genuinely beautiful and exhibits
examples of occasional realistic observation. This multicolored blackberry is a particularly pleas-
ing example of the artist's skill. By permission of the Bodleian Library, Ms. 130, fo. 26.

These same books were frequently copied together, but the Bury copy of the Apuleius herbal was extraordinarily fine. Many depictions of flowers, leaves, and roots had become increasingly stylized over the centuries, losing any vital realistic detail; but of the 141 specimens sketched in this copy, some 21 were expertly drawn from life and correctly labeled. Pictures of the bramble, ground ivy, henbane, yarrow, hue, and cannabis were particularly well executed. Since some of the plants were not indigenous to Britain, they were presumably cultivated in the Bury herb garden and there studied by the artist. Such naturalism in scientific art was unanticipated in earlier works and would again lapse after 1150 as artists, hagiographers, and historians left concrete detail and returned to more schematic conventions. The Bury herbal continued to be used for the next two centuries, and notes were made in the margins adding the English equivalents of the Latin plant names.[13]

At the opposite end of the scale were the completely fanciful books. Early in the twelfth century, for example, another collection was transcribed and illustrated, this time in a pocket-sized version. The contents included a calendar, a treatise on the heavenly bodies complete with the signs of the zodiac and a picture of an astronomer with his astrolabe, and an ancient, untitled tract now called the *Marvels of the East*. Its plants, animals, and naked beings were depicted in such perennial fantasies as gem trees, unicorns, satyrs, and storks. Contemporary curiosities such as parrots and cannibals mixed company with headless, two-faced, or animal-topped men, with bearded, cloven-footed, tailed women, with hermaphrodites, and with outsized double-headed monsters. Grotesque creatures had always been familiar in the repertoire of Celtic art, but this booklet treated them as marvels, not merely as sinuous, decorative forms.[14]

Far more significant than this solitary collection, which apparently had no direct descendants, were the popular moralized natural histories now called bestiaries. Profusely illustrated, these books were ultimately based upon an ancient Greek work called the *Physiologus*, but their more direct antecedents included early Christian tracts, some possibly by the hermits of Egypt. In the early twelfth century bestiaries experienced a sudden renaissance, expanding in size and scope and becoming an almost uniquely English literary phenomenon. In alphabetical order they set out the names, habits, and symbolic Christian interpretations of animals and birds, real and imagined. Descriptions of the magical, medical, and symbolic properties of stones — lapidaries — were often attached. They, too, became more medically valuable at the end of the eleventh century and were markedly more popular in England than on the continent.[15]

Bestiaries had a split personality. They were at once fanciful picture books, important dictionaries of symbols, and critical catalogs of animal lore. Amidst a plethora of misconstrued behavior, illogical conjecture, and belabored etymologies; they often included accurate anatomical renderings

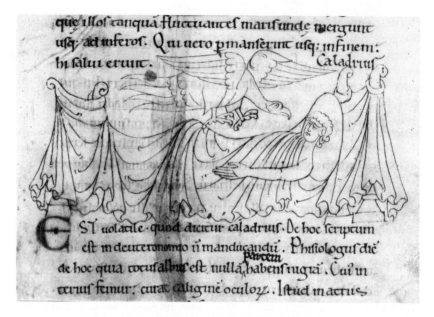

que illof tanquam fluctuancef marifunde mergunt
ufq; ad inferof. Qui uero pmanferint ufq; infinem:
hi falui erunt.   *Caladriuf*

EST uolatile · quod dicitur caladriuf. De hoc fcriptum
eft in deuteronomio ñ manducandu. Phifiologuf dic̄
de hoc quia totuf albuf eft nulla habenf rugia. Cui in
teriuf femur: curat caligine oculoꝝ. Iftud in actuẽ

THE CALADRIUS PREDICTS RECOVERY

The legendary caladrius was a favorite subject in medical books. Immaculately white, the bird represented prognostication and, when it inclined toward a patient, miraculous cure. This earliest example dates from 1120x1130 and is from an elaborate, illustrated bestiary, which is itself the oldest English specimen of that strange blend of naturalistic, fantastic, and symbolic literature. Other sketches in this manuscript, like the pigeon on fo. 161, are quite realistic. By permission of the Bodleian Library, Ms. Laud 247, fo. 142.

of familiar species and precise details of zoological study. Never noted for their literary merit, they nonetheless mirrored the contemporary mixture of allegory and observation.

Typical of the whole genre is the discussion of the caladrius, Immaculately white, this long-necked bird hovers at the foot of a sick man's bed. The frightened patient stares at the visitor, knowing it is about to offer a prognosis of his illness. If the snow bird inclines in the man's direction, he will recover. If the caladrius turns away, the patient will die. Moreover, if the illness be not mortal, the bird can take upon himself the whole infirmity of the man, fly up toward the sun, and dissipate the sickness in the firy air. Would that all medical knowledge were so uncomplicated.

Although the caladrius could and did symbolize Christ taking upon Himself the sins of humanity, its earlier manifestations can be traced back through Pliny to Plato and beyond. Centuries later, the mythical bird was still a common image in Norman Britain. It was illustrated in bestiaries and medical treatises, described in works of theology, and even carved on parish walls, such as those of the church at Alne in Yorkshire.[16] One of the few medical symbols ever so honored, the bird and the bestiaries themselves were particularly popular in the north of England. The white caladrius suggests the search of medieval people, and of all people, for health, for foreknowledge, and for miraculous cure.

Bestiaries, lapidaries, and herbals—in effect, rudimentary animal, mineral, and vegetable studies—spoke more to the general fascination with strange marvels than to the details of medical practice. There were, however, many pragmatic manuals. Sometimes sets of prescriptions came in full treatises, but more often a few pages of medical recipes and antidotes were copied on blank pages of completely unrelated volumes.[17] The larger miscellanies were often revised and new drugs were even added. For surgical techniques, the manuscript illustrations, such as sketches of delicate eye operations and incisions for nasal polyps and hemorrhoids, often prove more informative than the accompanying texts. One of the most familiar subjects, a naked man being prepared for cauterization, bridged studies of anatomy and surgery; black dots on his body pinpointed the best places to apply the burning iron.[18]

At the end of the eleventh century other books began to filter into Britain, particularly from workshops in Salerno. These new studies, really long-lost sections of works by famous authors like Hippocrates and Galen, had been preserved in the Islamic East. After 1077, many such texts were translated from Arabic back into Latin by a converted Moslem, an enterprising former merchant called Constantine the African. They dealt with the general responsibilities of physicians and with particular topics like fever, urinalysis, and surgery. Although the subjects Constantine selected sound quite clinical, he usually translated the most theoretical parts rather than complete works. Theory was especially prevalent in treatises that emphasized the role of astrology in medicine. For some men celestial computation became an important part of forecasting the possibility of a cure and the best time for treatment. On a more practical level, such texts at least increased the body of information that could be conveniently taught in schools to large groups of students.

On the other hand, much truly valid wisdom silently passed from master to disciple without ever touching the written page. Old books, after all, are only dim reflectors of real life, and the few existing compilations certainly do not exhaust English knowledge of the art of medicine.[19] Unduly emphasizing them or segregating medicine from other studies can distort the past. Anglo-Norman people were curious about many things. Although they loved to devise elaborate charts outlining the various branches of knowledge, they were not enamored of rigid specialization. Every learned man self-confidently believed he should know something about medicine, as well as theology and canon law—the three so-called practical sciences. The fre-

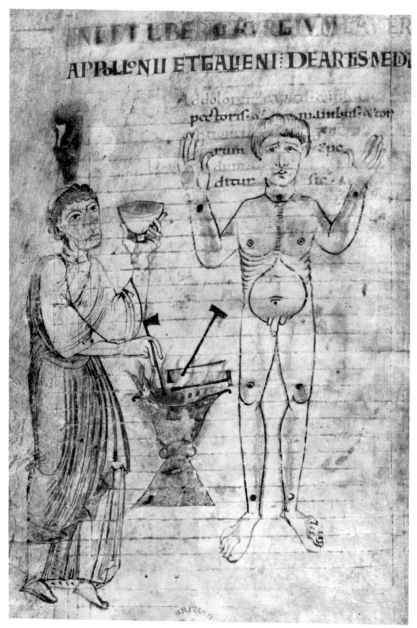

EARLY CAUTERIZATION

Four pages of these naked, rather realistic cautery men were drawn about 1100 to accompany a small, pocket-sized collection of medical tracts. Cauterization was applied to many conditions, including the elephantiasis and rectal complaints illustrated on another page. The inscription

quent library mixture of bestiaries, herbals, surgical treatises, and astronomical tables bears witness to this view of life. As laymen studied medicine, so many physicians equally considered themselves poets, historians, and statesmen.

Readers of the literature of medicine and marvels were far more numerous than the naturalists who wrote the books, but the authors had considerable influence. They can now be divided into four types, but as generalists, they themselves would undoubtedly have resisted categorization. Although most naturalists were too isolated for committee meetings or cooperative projects, they did often conquer poor communications and long distances to keep abreast of their colleagues' publications.

The first large, rather passive, group has already been mentioned. Its members comprised the anonymous copyists, mainly Saxon monks, who diligently transcribed bestiaries, herbals, and marvels. They were intrigued by natural phenomena, but they recorded what others thought about it rather than offer new insights. Although the works of the copyists lacked originality, their choices determined what people read. The increasing accuracy of their sketches has been noted, as has their eventual change from Saxon studies to translated Arabic sources. Meticulous research has now localized their activity to certain great monasteries, such as Worcester, Thorney, Hereford, Peterborough, and Saint Augustine's Canterbury, all strongholds of Saxon culture.[20]

Versatile amateurs make up the second group. Often born of mixed Norman-Saxon parentage, they were directly engaged in the present but equally in love with the past. Many were historians who recorded unusual natural occurrences as frequently as contemporary political events. For example, John of Worcester chronicled his own times and also studied astronomy, noted celestial changes, and transcribed the latest writings of men like Adelard of Bath and Honorius of Autun. Henry of Huntingdon, a secular clerk and busy archdeacon, composed poetry and historical narrative, and also wrote, or copied, a lapidary and a herbal, and composed works on miracles and weights and measures.[21]

William of Malmesbury best typifies this mentality. His parents sent him at an early age to Malmesbury Abbey, the shrine of a great Saxon saint, Aldhelm. Although this Wiltshire monastery was an undistinguished place during much of its history, it did attract some unusual monks. Long before William's time a brother named Elmer had glued wings to his back and jumped from the church belfry. Although crippled by the crash, this medi-

---

reads, "Here begins Appollonius's Book of Surgery and Cautery and Galen's Art of Medicine. For aching head, flatulence of breast and hands, and pain of knees and feet, burn thus." Such figures with application points clearly marked on their bodies frequently served as medical illustrations. By permission of the British Library, Ms. Sloane 2839, fo. 1.

eval Daedalus always claimed it was his own fault for forgetting to add a tail! Elmer apparently wrote some minor astronomical tracts and later, in 1066, as a very old man watching Haley's comet, he claimed he remembered its earlier visitation in 989. The abbey also housed world travelers. In 1102–3 a merchant named Saewulf went to Jerusalem. Shortly thereafter he joined the abbey and wrote a short guidebook to the places he had seen. Three famous physicians, Faritius, Gregory, and Robert de Venys, were associated with Malmesbury, and William's own mentor, Abbot Godfrey, greatly expanded its library.[22]

The range of William's reading was extraordinary, probably the widest of his time.[23] In an interesting reference to his education the monk noted that he preferred studying medicine to logic but that his favorites were ethics and history.[24] The identity of William's medical instructor remains elusive; his interests seem akin to those of Faritius, but Gregory fits the time frame a little better. William knew not only the great books of theology and classical literature but also the latest works on the abacus, on Arabic culture and medicine, calendrical and chronological problems, astronomy, and the bestiary.[25] He traveled the length of the country for his careful documentary research and made personal observations about topography, ancient monuments, and the physical appearance of certain individuals. Both this careful investigation and his penchant for continually revising his writing reflect his delight in precise detail.

Beginning before 1118 and continuing for the next quarter century, William produced theological and exegetical tracts, saints' lives, monographs on certain religious houses, and major studies of the English church and government. Several manuscripts in his hand still exist. Some are drafts of his own compositions; others are his copies of colleagues' books. He knew the works of contemporaries like Honorius of Autun and Hildebert of Lavardin and was personally acquainted with writers of the stature of John of Worcester and important patrons such as Queen Matilda.

Chroniclers like William were somewhat ambivalent about health care. On the one hand, they proudly paraded their own medical knowledge, recorded symptoms, and offered diagnoses. On the other, they devoutly attributed significant healing to God and believed that He frequently intervened in human affairs to cure individuals. Their writing is filled with accounts of sufferers wasting their coin on useless medical treatments before being miraculously cured through the intercession of a saint. William, in particular, seldom missed a chance to demonstrate the greed of physicians.[26] Interestingly, such repeated condemnations also show the accessibility of medical care and the high regard average folk had for it. Most people lived in two worlds—time and spirit—and saw no contradiction in seeking the remedies of both.

In addition to the scribes and amateurs there was a group of naturalists, the new pioneers—men actually involved in scientific and technical progress. Many were foreigners or Englishmen who had studied abroad. They show up in the church, the government, and in ordinary society. Sometimes they were quite pragmatic, less interested in ultimate causes or strange appearances than in how things worked. A clear mathematical base supported all their efforts. They analyzed chronological computation, the effect of weather on human life, and the problems of stone vault construction. Their greatest success lay in popularizing the abacus method of calculation; the royal bureaucracy quickly adapted this to splendid use at the exchequer. Two immigrants from Lorraine, Robert the bishop of Hereford (d. 1095), and Walcher the prior of Malvern (d. 1125), wrote about the abacus, as did the famed Adelard of Bath and an obscure man named Turkill, probably an exchequer clerk active before 1115.[27] The new development of this ancient apparatus spotlights an important aspect of Anglo-Norman science, a very real commitment to solving contemporary problems. The age-old Christian study of chronology, after all, sprang from a continual need to recalculate the moveable feast of Easter.

Sometimes the investigators stood on the very frontiers of knowledge. Astronomy was especially attractive, and twelfth-century stargazers carefully observed the heavens and recorded their findings, often with the aid of another newly popular mechanism, the astrolabe. Their mentality was radically different from that of the scribes or versatile amateurs. Intolerant of traditional Western concepts, they were obsessed with mastering the learning of the East and set about obtaining all the Arabic and Greek translations available. To a limited extent they also tried—or at least preached—original experimentation. Adelard was the most obvious exponent of this viewpoint, but he was undoubtedly influenced by Pedro Alfonso, King Henry's converted Jewish physician from Spain.

Pedro brings the circuit back not only to the royal court but also to the last group, the professional practitioners—those architects, engineers, and physicians who directly employed the new learning. In medicine there were several levels of performance. Countless practitioners of folk medicine used the tried and true remedies of experience. Superstitious tribal memory sometimes influenced their judgment, but so did keen insight into human psychology. Paraprofessional practitioners, such as midwives, hospital masters, and bleeders, were on another tier. Phlebotomists, often later equated with barber-surgeons, do not appear this way in the early records. Scholastic practitioners—regular professors of medicine—exulted in a higher position, but their influence has probably been overemphasized.

Amidst all this stood the actual physician, the medicus. He was a general practitioner rather than a specialist, and the distinction between physician and surgeon was not yet very meaningful. Englishmen may have obtained medical education at academic centers such as Chartres, Montpellier, and

Salerno. Certainly, British attendance at these schools increased in the course of the century. Apprentice doctors with fewer financial resources undoubtedly learned their trade at home in direct experience with patients. However, no full-fledged medical school can be reliably identified in early twelfth-century Britain.

Some aspects of Anglo-Norman practice have an unexpectedly modern flavor. Pills were already known, and there were even tentative references to a type of early anesthesia.[28] Disease was thought to occur naturally, to be a part of life. Only very rarely were demons or sin diagnosed as the cause of illness, except occasionally for "leprosy." Even when people were thought to be cured miraculously, the process was seldom instantaneous. Those who recorded marvels seemed to appreciate the need for time, as well as for divine intervention, in such healings. Laws required that the insane be treated compassionately; one dour observer said that this should be truer "the more we understand that the human race grows sick with the harshness of a cruel fortune."[29] There were frequent reports of individuals cured of depression or fits of raving, but some violent people were tied down or otherwise forcibly restrained.

Hygiene may have been better than generally imagined. Monasteries installed elaborate indoor plumbing, as any visitor to an excavated cloister can attest. Abbot Ailred of Rievaulx was able to take as many as forty baths a day when tortured by bladder or kidney stones. Cleanliness, that is, bathing and washing, was a preferred treatment for many conditions. Even the contemporary master of romanic fiction, Geoffrey of Monmouth, praised the efficacy of bathing. In one of the earliest references to Stonehenge (which is also an interesting allusion to lapidary and herbal medicine), Geoffrey reported that people were cured in baths of herbal concoctions and water that had run over the medicinally potent stones.[30]

Archaeology reveals that episcopal and mercantile townhouses also boasted lead pipes and stone drains and that early urban dwellers carefully designed their wells and cesspits. Latrines were often neatly lined in wood or stone, periodically cleaned out, and carefully dug some distance from property boundaries. Perhaps some lost civic regulation directed the sanitary placement. A twelfth-century wooden toilet seat, latrine pit, and wicker screen for privacy were recently excavated in York. In Oxford there were even indoor toilets in basement cellars. Peasant and burgher houses were often swept quite clean, betraying none of the litter so often ascribed to them and so regularly uncovered on late Roman sites. Regretfully, conditions deteriorated as urban communities grew older and more crowded.[31]

The point at issue now, after this quick background tour through medical customs and literature, is what people were doing about health care. Did anyone take the lead in providing better service? In particular, what were the roles of the court and the church?

King Henry I (b. 1069, reigned 1100–35) was the towering personality of the age, and he affected almost every facet of English life, including health services. His successor, King Stephen (b. c. 1096, reigned 1135–54), was a fascinating failure of a man. Ineffective as a ruler, he also had only marginal medical interests. Together they presided over an era of immense change, sometimes bending it to their will, sometimes being overwhelmed by its force. For the most part Henry and his associates managed to keep the peace in England, though not in Normandy. Stephen quickly lost control of the duchy and suffered continuous rebellion in the home shires. Careful scholarship has significantly enlarged the portraits of these two unusual monarchs, but it has not yet defined all their social welfare policies.[32]

Resolute, inquisitive, and clever, Henry was a first-rate king but a rather unlikeable person. His lust was legendary, but his equally infamous cruelty and greed were probably directed by state policy as much as by individual perversity. Short, ruddy, and as he aged, fat and probably balding in the front, he was an unimposing figure but a dynamic leader. In his time government was an intensely personal operation and its staff, institutions, and scope were severely limited. Family, village, and feudal loyalties were often more important to people than was royal authority, and the sovereign frequently had to assert his rights against local resistance.

Henry therefore chose his advisers and deputies with exceptional care and was pleased when they made impressive strides in raising his administration to a more rational, multidimensional level. Naturally such ministers were most concerned about royal revenues, and they immediately took steps to create a stable, profitable financial order. Through experimentation the exchequer system was perfected, a bureaucracy established, and royal justice brought to more people. These innovations did not mature overnight, but most were evidently well under way in the first decade of the reign.

Demands of his troublesome duchy frequently called Henry across the Channel, and it eventually turned out that he had been physically present in Britain for less than half of his long thirty-five-year reign. Consequently much of the unacknowledged credit for his governmental reforms, and indeed for the general well-being of the whole realm, must go to his permanent counsellors, especially to his brilliant viceroy and lifelong executive, Bishop Roger of Salisbury.[33]

Fortunately, the king and his officials lived in an age when religious enthusiasm inspired people to extend themselves in concrete works of charity. Although he acted for his own reasons, Henry was exceptionally responsive to concerns of public welfare and the range of his provisions for commerce and education was unprecedented.[34] His interests in popular health care were equally unusual. They may have been stimulated by the spread of the sicknesses called leprosy and by other national calamities. Henry was terribly upset by multiple problems in 1130 and quite ill three years later, but he had been away from England for most of the earlier bad times. Therefore his initial concern was probably less a forced response to external events than a deep-seated personal commitment. This unique attachment seems to have been fostered by his two wives' many charities, his concept of public responsibility, his pleasure in strange marvels, and his desire for stimulating companionship.

King Henry's decision to include physicians in his retinue is hardly surprising. Since at least Edward the Confessor's time, English monarchs had regularly traveled with their personal medical attendants. Most of the known doctors of the Conqueror's era were monks, but physicians who accompanied him were probably secular clerks and laymen. William Rufus also kept his own doctors, but their names were not preserved. More extraordinary is the large number of physicians directly associated with King Henry. Eight such practitioners can be identified, many of whom gained substantial influence at court. (Their careers will be examined in Chapter 3). Ultimately Henry disregarded their sound dietary advice, but otherwise he held physicians in great regard. Constantly seeking their company, he richly rewarded their services and encouraged his family to develop similar relationships. Contrariwise, King Stephen appears to have had not even a single physician, but he and his wife did support several hospitals.

Henry's first consort, Matilda, the only Scottish princess ever to wed an English king, exerted a major influence on her husband. Originally named Edith, she was the daughter of King Malcolm Canmore (d. 1093) (the successor of Macbeth) and his beautiful Saxon queen, Margaret (d. 1093), a lady renowned throughout Christendom for her sanctity, charity, and artistic patronage. One of her good works was sponsorship of the great hospital of Saint Giles at Edinburgh.

After the death of her parents Edith—or Matilda, as the Normans invariably called her—was educated at an aristocratic Wessex nunnery and was soon more Norman in taste than Saxon or Scot. Through her mother, father, and husband, Matilda unified the Old English, Scottish, and Norman royal families and was thus the ideal bride for Henry, the usurper king. It was through her that not only Henry but all succeeding English kings achieved a bloodlink to the pre-Conquest dynasties of the island. Some question remained as to whether Matilda had actually taken the veil in the convent, but nonetheless, within three months of Henry's seizure of his slain brother's throne she had become queen.[35]

Matilda's priceless lineage guaranteed her significant independence in the conduct of her affairs. Henry seems to have respected and trusted her, even if his roaming lust and her less-than-passionate attention denied them a life of amorous intimacy. Matilda gave birth to three children. At age twenty-one, in 1101, she was assisted in her first confinement by two eminent Italian physicians, Faritius abbot of Abingdon and his lay colleague, Grimbald. The baby, perhaps named Richard, died in infancy. A daughter, Matilda, grew to become empress of the Holy Roman Empire, unsuccessful opponent of King Stephen, and mother of Henry II of England. In 1103 a boy, William, a frail child destined to tragedy, entered the world. The monastic chronicler William of Malmesbury, who knew both the doctors and the queen herself, was singularly restrained in his praise of her and rather cryptically noted that, having had a child of either sex, Matilda considered her duty done and had no more.[36]

She seems to have found compensation in government, literature, and charity. Although making at least three trips to Normandy with her husband, she occasionally remained behind as regent. Matilda then threw herself into the administrative routine of hearing pleas and issuing writs. Most of the cases brought before her concerned lands where she already had a personal interest. Even then, her decisions were usually made in concert with Roger of Salisbury, the real head of the government under the king.[37] On the whole, Matilda was more interested in establishing policies than in executing them. She liked to begin things and normally moved directly, even brusquely, to her objective.

Her correspondence reflected a wide, although perhaps not deep, acquaintance with several eminent thinkers, including the reforming pope, Paschal II, the exiled archbishop, Anselm of Canterbury, and the three poet-prelates, Hildebert of Lavardin, Baudri of Bourgueil and Ivo of Chartres. She was an active champion of foreign bards, favoring sweet-voiced minstrels, but her patronage of them was so extravagant that it caused genuine concern and expense to her tenants. They were strong-minded people themselves and not backward in complaining about her exactions. Besides theology, poetry, and music, Matilda was also interested in biography, history, and romance. She commissioned a Latin life of her holy mother from one author, Turgot, and urged another, William of Malmesbury, to explain the history of the English kings.[38]

A man named Benedict prepared for her an Anglo-Norman French translation of the *Voyage of Saint Brendan*, the adventures of a sixth-century Irish traveler. This early example of the gentry vernacular further popularized miracles, wonders, and geographical curiosities. When describing the walls of paradise, the translator inserted a long discussion of precious stones—a regular miniature lapidary—(absent from the original tale). Icebergs, volcanos, walruses, dragons, griffins, and whales carrying men on their backs were all part of this amusing tale of a transatlantic voyage westward to a new world. This narrative shares certain features with the ancient eastern story of Sinbad the sailor but also typifies the English—and the universal—passion for exotic knowledge.[39]

Most of all, Matilda was remembered for her good works. She witnessed the reburial of Saxon relics, took a special interest in the cult of Saint Mary

Magdalene, washed the feet of lepers, and supposedly wore a hair shirt. Early in the reign her husband gave her the collegiate church of Waltham Holy Cross in Essex, a renowned center for educators, writers, and medical men. From the canons she drew some of her personal staff; other followers were rewarded with benefices. Monasteries such as Durham, which had its own connections with Waltham, and Tynemouth, Westminster, and Romsey also enjoyed her favor, but above all she was active in establishing houses for the recently founded order of Austin canons. These men were more directly involved in social work than the monks, especially in the rising towns. In exchange for certain of its London properties, Waltham once received a watermill from the queen. She then used the city tenements to endow the Austin priory of Holy Trinity, Aldgate.[40]

Several of Matilda's projects touched public welfare even more directly. She built at least two stone bridges in the Essex countryside. In London, not far from Saint Paul's Cathedral, at her large riverside wharf called Queenhithe, she erected one of the city's first public lavatories. Presumably this was a rather elaborate bath complex.[41] Following the lead of her mother, she also began to build hospitals. Her major foundation was the large leprosarium, Saint Giles-in-the Fields, at Holborn, just outside the twelfth-century limits of the city of London. A much smaller facility, Saints James and Mary Magdalene, was raised at Chichester. These creations and her further interests in leper care will be more fully discussed when all the Henrican hospitals are examined in Chapter 4. It is worth remembering at the outset, however, that her example encouraged the king and several bishops and barons to undertake similar large-scale works of mercy.

The queen was only in her late thirties when she died in 1118. Henry was abroad, but at his order she was buried next to the Confessor in Westminster Abbey, rather than at Holy Trinity as she had wished. Maud lacked favor with contemporary monastic writers, who evidently never forgave her for leaving the convent, but the common people felt differently. One hundred and fifty years after her death she was still praised for directing public opinion to a more charitable attitude toward lepers. Miracles were occasionally attributed to her intercession, but she was never canonized.[42]

In 1120 Matilda and Henry's son, William, the hope of their dynasty, perished miserably in the wreck of the *White Ship*. A year later Henry took a second bride, the singularly beautiful Adeliza of Louvain, whose own lineage could be traced back to Charlemagne. Although Henry had numerous illegitimate offspring, and although Adeliza would have seven children by a second marriage, no issue blessed this union. Adeliza cultivated many of Matilda's other interests, however. Copies of the *Voyage of Saint Brendan* were redidicated to the new queen, and she asked a writer named David to compose a history of Henry's reign.

Adeliza evidently enjoyed the company of physicians. One medicus,

Master Serlo of Arundel, who was associated with the Waltham canons and who may have come from there himself, remained with her for more than fifteen years. Another physician, Robert, had a less important place in her retinue. Adeliza also founded hospitals of her own. One was courteously situated at Wilton where Queen Matilda had once been educated. It, too, was dedicated to Saint Giles, the patron of lepers.

Another writer Adeliza sponsored was Philip de Thaon, a Waltham canon. He knew Turkill's work on the abacus and was familiar with Brendan's story about the sleeping whale. Before 1120 he had already prepared a somewhat clumsy treatise for priests, which explained the astronomical, chronological, and calendrical rules for determining the correct date of Easter. For the new queen, Philip composed a bestiary and a rather symbolistic, or allegorical lapidary. It has been called an apocalyptic lapidary because, somewhat like Benedict in the tale of Brendan, Philip treats the twelve foundation stones of the heavenly Jerusalem. A second, more medical, discussion of stones by Philip found its way into the library of Doctor Herbert of Durham. In his bestiary Canon Philip included the caladrius, but added the unusual details that the white bird had a thigh bone of great size and that a salve from its marrow could restore sight to a blind man.

Despite such flights of fancy, Philip's works were not usually very original, and the extant copies of his bestiary have blank spaces where the miniatures should have been painted. On the other hand, he wrote in the Anglo-Norman vernacular and employed a metrical form with such poetic devices as the octosyllabic rhyming couplet. Dull, pedantic, and well-meaning, the canon recorded provincial, outdated science, but he did create an important linguistic monument. His selections also demonstrate that the royal family's reading habits paralleled the general scientific interests of the country.[43]

Henry loved marvels as much as his wives did. A strange chalice found in an ancient graveyard was sent to the king and the circumstances of its recovery were carefully noted. Tales of green-colored children, deformed animals, and odd celestial occurrences were reported to the court. Henry even kept a large menagerie of exotic animals—a regular zoo—at Woodstock Palace. Suppliants and visitors soon learned that one of the best ways to gain royal attention was to bring some rare specimen—a falcon, a polar bear, or maybe even an elephant. William of Malmesbury reported seeing a camel, an ostrich, and a porcupine there.[44]

Henry's lifelong fascination with prophecy was also notorious. Indeed, at the end, Matilda's mother had been as much given to prediction as had the king's own father. Both had prophesied that their children would be sovereigns, a most unlikely prospect at the moment of the pronouncements.[45] Contemporary writers such as William of Malmesbury, Ordericus Vitalis, Geoffrey of Monmouth, and Abbot Suger in France recorded other predictions about the king.

In particular there was the famous old prophecy of the dying King Edward, which forecast that England would not prosper again until a green tree was cut down, replanted, and regenerated. A twelfth-century medical manuscript even had a recipe for reuniting a split green rod.[46] The favored interpretation cast Henry's son, William the Atheling, as the fulfillment of the dream but it was not to be. After the prince's drowning in 1120 the king still sought to learn the future and even personally consulted the hermit physician and prophet, Wulfric of Haselbury. In fact, making prophecies, recording miracles, studying astronomy, and practicing medicine frequently went together and, early and late, Henry surrounded himself with men who possessed one or more of these talents.

Indeed, the king may even have thought that he, personally, enjoyed medical powers. The evidence is undeniably weak, but there were contemporary rumors that kings could heal certain illnesses. During his reign people in France and England were increasingly convinced that one monarchial attribute was thaumaturgic power, sometimes dubbed the royal touch. Supposedly, anointed rulers in those countries could miraculously cure jaundice, leprosy, or scrofula. Although not always precisely distinguished and occasionally even confused with simple swellings and running sores, one or another of these repulsive maladies at various times was called the *morbus regis*, which has been translated as the royal disease or sickness, or even more dramatically, as the king's evil. To the classical Romans the term meant jaundice. From the patristic age through the twelfth century it also generally denoted leprosy. Thereafter it referred to scrofula. The foundations of the puzzling belief that medieval kings could heal such disease are difficult to pin down, but the assertion bedeviled much of later European history.[47]

King Henry's own involvement in this curious practice was far more speculative than that of his fellow sovereigns. In France miraculous healing has been tentatively ascribed to Robert the Pious (reigned 996 – 1031) and was considered hereditary in the Capetian dynasty from Philip I (reigned 1060–1108) onward. In England the situation was quite ambiguous. Edward the Confessor reportedly healed sufferers both as an exile in Normandy and, afterwards, at home as king of the Saxons. Thus his curing seemed to stem from personal sanctity rather than from consecrated royalty.

The Confessor was canonized in 1163, almost a full century after his death. In the intervening years several propagandists actively promoted his cause. About 1080 the Flemish hack writer, Goscelin of Saint Bertin, was employed by Edward's widow to explain the king's life and certify his miracles. In the next generation sympathetic local monks, like William of Malmesbury and Osbert of Clare, taxed their pens in his behalf. In one of Goscelin's stories a married but barren woman with a severe case of swollen neck glands dreamed that she had been commanded to have the king wash them. Edward did eventually bathe and massage her neck until all sorts of putrid matter poured forth. He comforted her at his court as the wound healed during the following week. Presumably the woman lived happily ever after; at any rate, she soon had twins! Oddly enough, the king's therapy resembled that of a regular physician rather than that of a faith healer.

However, others besides Edward were said to cure the king's evil. Goscelin reported that Saint Edith (d. 984) healed a severe eye disorder, which he called the royal sickness. On the other hand, William of Malmesbury always identified the royal disease exclusively with leprosy. For example, saintly Wulfstan of Worcester (d. 1095) once unintentionally healed such a case. A stricken pauper was horribly wasting away, but he managed to travel cross-country from Kent to Worcester to beg the bishop's aid. Wulfstan treated him charitably, but did not think he could help. Fortunately, two members of his household, Elmer and Arthur, took pity on the leper's distress, craftily smuggled out water in which Wulfstan had washed his hands after Mass, and poured it into the sick man's bath. When the suppliant lowered himself into the water, his sores melted away.

In later ages, when saints were no longer personally available, their relics sometimes sufficed. For example, the bones of Saint Milburga (d. 715) were rediscovered in 1101 and quickly became famed for their effect on lepers, victims of the royal disease, which William said doctors could not cure.[48]

Unquestionably, ardent faith brought some sick persons temporary remission or permanent cure of their ailments. The question is, How much did King Edward's successors promote this effort? Some modern historians think William the Conqueror may have "touched" for serious complaints, but others reject such early usage.[49] In fact, the practice was not formally ascribed to any English prince after Edward until Henry II. It is thus doubtful that King Henry I ever publicly acknowledged such thaumaturgic power, but he was far too pragmatic to deny the advantage of having others believe it.

One of William of Malmesbury's anecdotes certainly suggests this probability. About 1125, in his own version of the Confessor's cure of the barren woman afflicted with swollen glands, the monk added an important, if rather snappish, observation to Goscelin's account. William reported that reliable witnesses still testified that even before Edward was crowned he had performed such miracles in exile. Therefore it should be obvious, he said, that "today some men set out to deceive by asserting that the power to cure that sort of disease is not the product of holiness, but an hereditary royal prerogative."[50] This rather convoluted remark is authentic but oblique testimony to the strength of a popular belief the chronicler himself deplored. William felt that only true saints could perform miracles. His intent was to deny a contemporary rumor about King Edward, not to examine the practice of King Henry. Nevertheless, the monk's very rejection demonstrates that some subjects of Henry felt that their king, simply because he was king, could heal disease.

It is worth considering why Henry may have desired such distinction. He was hardly a saintly man, but he did grow increasingly devout as his years multiplied. More to the point, he was acutely sensitive of his own prerogatives, real or imagined. Even before his coronation Henry had worked out a theory of his own unique throne-worthiness: he claimed the crown by porphyrogeniture. That is, he alone of William of Normandy's sons was born after the Conquest and thus only he was the son of a king, born in and to the purple. Furthermore, like his father and his brother, he described himself as the heir of King Edward, but only his descent was confirmed in marriage. Even death strengthened the connection. In 1102 Edward's tomb at Westminster was opened and his body found incorrupt. Sixteen years later Henry insisted that his wife Maud be interred right next to the Confessor.

Besides this borrowed glory, other factors may have urged Henry to encourage his subjects to think of him as a prince-physician. Accepting the role required no medical training, but it could counterbalance a French king's pretensions. Moreover, in the wake of compromise with the pope, Henry probably welcomed any posture that restored a spiritual dimension to his kingship.[51]

Early in his reign Henry and Archbishop Anselm had quarreled over the papacy's reform program. In particular, the king wished to maintain royal control over the selection of church officials and the associated symbolic investiture of their benefices. He agreed to settle the controversy only when he began to conquer Normandy in the guise of a protector of its troubled church. Although still demanding feudal homage from ecclesiastical vassals, Henry did relinquish the practice of investing them with ring and crozier. He thereby surrendered his dynasty's claim to theocratic, quasi-priestly rule.

Lacking this hereditary sacral prerogative, Henry may well have tried to repaint something of his spiritual lineaments by tolerating an existing belief that he, as king, could heal leprosy. Accordingly, his special patronage of leper hospitals may indeed have been a concrete and more beneficial expression of this same attitude. Perhaps he reasoned that leprosy, as the so-called royal disease, particularly deserved his personal compassion.

King Henry apparently accepted miracles as readily as everyone else. He, too, coveted holy relics and even obtained the arm of Saint James the Greater for the new royal monastery at Reading. Although often tight-fisted, he could lavish gifts upon certain religious houses and liberally donate to the poor. He was not immune to the beneficial influence of associates who included both talented civil servants and quite spiritually minded men.

Henry's court encouraged an unusual array of contending forces. Besides the normal conferences about military preparedness, judicial administration, financial solvency, political patronage, and church appointments, it is reasonable to imagine that there must have been many lengthy discussions about the virulence of leprosy, the importance of Arabic learning, the use of

the abacus, the meaning of animal symbolism, the purpose of different vocations, and the effectiveness of charitable assistance. Similar debates
evidently took place in other parts of the country. The argument is indeed
circular: royal interest helped multiply the numbers of doctors, hospitals,
and medical books, and this expansion gave health care a higher governmental priority than it might otherwise have enjoyed.

The outstanding administrative innovations of the reign, the king's rather
repugnant personal qualities, the constant movement of the royal court, the
foreign wars, the conflicting ambitions of barons, and the lengthy quarrel
with the church over investitures—all of these factors hide the genuine
spiritual revival Henry's age experienced. Surely one barometer of that religious enthusiasm was the steady stream of curial officials who became hermits, monks, and canons. Further effects of the king's religious interests, his
possible thaumaturgic claims, the charity and patronage of his wives, and
the general delight in marvels can be demonstrated by the royal family's impressive sponsorship of hospital facilities and continuous association with a
large corps of diversified physicians.

First, however, a final word should be said of the related attitude of the
church to social welfare. Three misconceptions have unnecessarily distorted
the straightforward record of ecclesiastical support for health care. First, it
has been claimed that the church opposed all medical practice because it
fundamentally abhorred the shedding of human blood. Second, some commentators have declared that the hierarchy forbade its priests and religious
to act as physicians. Third, it has been said that clerical establishments were
concerned about the physical health of only their own members and that
monastic physicians and abbey hospitals therefore catered exclusively to fellow religious. None of these interpretations depict the reality of Anglo-
Norman conditions.

The contention that the church detested any shedding of human blood
was undoubtedly true as an aphorism and as an injunction against hatred
and war, but it had no medical significance. Indeed, the statement cannot
be found in any early ecclesiastical decree. Its frequent citation in modern
textbooks has no basis in medieval fact and seems to arise from an eighteenth-
century hoax.[52] On the other hand, when the Gregorian reformers decided
to reorder the spiritual and political priorities of their world, they did set in
motion a thorough examination of the duties of all Christians. The hierarchy
that finally emerged from this renewal was extremely concerned about how
its ministers understood their calling. Thus a number of local and universal
church councils attacked as unseemly the joint vocation of monk and physician.

In 1123, for example, the First Lateran Council forbade monks to visit the
sick (*infirmos visitare*). But what did this mean? Like any phrase, the words
had both a literal meaning and a pertinent context. The associated regula-

tions reveal that the fathers were not condemning medical treatment, or even such practice by monks, but, rather, lucrative rewards and improper worldly involvement. Medical service was not even the main thrust of the directive. The specific prohibition was part of a larger decree against monks giving public penances, consecrating altars, or ordaining clerics. It was intended to encourage them to lead more cloistered lives by denying them pastoral responsibilities. Regional councils, at Clermont in 1130 and Rheims in 1132, later forbade monks and regular canons, but not secular clerics, to study medicine or law for the sake of temporal gain. More important, in 1139 these condemnations were promulgated for the whole church at the Second Lateran Council. The effect of any of this legislation within England was problematical.[53]

Some chroniclers consistently satirized the greed and apparent uselessness of physicians, but such unsystematic hostility appears throughout history. In the New Testament, for example, the Evangelist Mark describes a woman who had been hemorrhaging for twelve years. She also had suffered much from doctors and "spent all her substance" on them without ever being helped; only when she came to Jesus was she cured. Later miracle stories have parallel episodes. William of Malmesbury even used a similar grammatical construction — she spent all her substance — to describe a Norman woman who turned from useless medical treatment to heavenly cure.[54] Despite the implied moral, such instances were never able to dictate formal church policy or popular religious belief. They were too easily countered by the well-known portrait of the Evangelist Luke as a skilled physician.

One anecdote can exemplify the different problems a monastic physician faced when treating lay patients. This account comes from the Continent, but the absence of pertinent English examples does not necessarily mean that England escaped the problem. Shortly before 1123 a doctor from the small Norman abbey of Flaix ran away to enter the Cistercian monastery of Clairvaux, complaining that his abbot had forced him to practice medicine for the benefit of others. Bernard of Clairvaux and the abbot of Flaix exchanged heated letters about the refugee who, according to canon law, clearly belonged in his original abbey. The difficulty was not in the abbot greedily abusing the man's talents to raise money but rather in his callously forcing this one monk to defend the privileges of the whole community. The barons in the area were a turbulent lot, and the abbot sought to keep them at bay by offering needed medical care. The monk had called the laity he unwillingly attended "tyrants, thieves, and excommunicates" and claimed that he helped them at the peril of his soul. Obviously the abbot thought this was an exaggeration. He probably felt that the doctor's worry was a small price to pay for the security of the whole monastery.[55]

Certainly there was an inherent tension, maybe even a contradiction, between the ideals of selfless withdrawal from the world and active involvement in contemporary affairs. Bernard of Clairvaux is himself a colossal example of a man who preached isolation and lived engagement. Nevertheless, the issue is not how individual men understood or rationalized their callings, but what the standard of the teaching church was. Here the lesson seems clear: help those in need, but do not profit from their distress. The forward movement of theological debate wished monks to follow their rules more precisely, but it never urged them to abandon medical knowledge. Certainly Anglo-Norman events refute any assertion that the twelfth-century church neglected the sick.

The English clergy was noticeably less interested in the speculations of theology and canon law than its continental counterparts, but it was equally affected by the pervasive influence of Christian reform. In the same years that hospital facilities, medical books, and identifiable physicians were so rapidly multiplying, the numbers of monastic houses and religious men and women were simultanously increasing eight times over. New orders, like the strict Cistercians and the civic-minded Austin canons, attracted many recruits, but the traditional Black Monk abbeys also grew in membership and possessions. The regular clergy, which staffed many of the cathedrals and most of the parish churches, also flourished.

Church leadership had become largely Norman or European since the Conquest, but thousands of Saxons continued to become priests, monks, nuns, canons, and lay brothers. Others sought salvation not only apart from the world but far beyond the formal patterns of organized religious societies. These hermits and anchorites, many of whom were women, were extremely important in rural life and performed all sorts of social services, such as keeping bridges in repair, teaching school, and safeguarding personal valuables, in addition to attending to their private devotions. Far from being distant, difficult world-weary recluses, the friendly neighborhood hermits were a common sight and valued community fixture. They were unusually inventive people and their unorganized activity often gave impetus to later, more systematized, institutions. Many twelfth century monasteries, schools, and hospitals could trace their origins to the experimental work of some socially minded solitary.

The hermits had informal allies in the colleges of secular canons that provided many of the same services in villages and small towns. Many canons, like Master Adelard of the college of Waltham Holy Cross, a noted educator and physician, were married. This made them unpopular with church reformers, but it did not stop such enthusiasts from readily copying their good ideas about social service. Since hermits and canons lacked any organized national fellowship or continuing group identity, few contemporary historians memorialized their collective achievements. They were, however, acutely attuned to local needs.

For a few years in the early twelfth century, old and new church institutions cooperated and competed. Many of the hidden springs of ecclesiastical and spiritual renewal bubbled up quite independently of any higher, or international, direction, but the streams of papal, episcopal, monastic and parish community reforms frequently converged. This enthusiasm was visible in the rush to Saxon hermitages, the creation of towering ecclesiastical buildings, the popularity of hagiographical scholarship, and, yes, the extended provision for health care.

The time has come, however, to turn from general environmental conditions, herbal traditions, royal pretensions, and ecclesiastical debates to the actual people who practiced medicine in Anglo-Norman England.

II. ANGLO-NORMAN PRACTITIONERS: A COMPOSITE PORTRAIT

People, not policies, create progress. The outgrowth of King Henry's fondness for miracles, marvels, and medicine and his sporadic interest in public welfare projects would have been frustrated had not a large, able corps of physicians and health care personnel shared his concerns. Awareness of the corporate existence and individual identity of these healers has long since faded, but they were once important community servants and faithful medical practitioners. Their significance deserves renewed recognition.

The medical achievements of Henry's reign, like his success in so many fields, arose partly from royal encouragement and partly from shrewd use of subordinates' talents, but the king rode the crest of a wave far beyond his full control. In a veritable groundswell, all ranks of society began to demand better social services, and by a happy coincidence, they also willingly developed the means to provide such care. Henry could, and did, capitalize on these powerful forces, but the physicians and the populace seem to have been quite capable of proceeding about their own good works without him.

Three questions immediately spring to mind. How large was that assembly of medical practitioners? Who were its members? What can be said about them? The queries are important, but none has an easy answer. This is somewhat surprising because Anglo-Norman England had an unsurpassed thirst for concrete statistical knowledge. Domesday Book epitomizes this yearning, but it is only the greatest of a whole series of detailed surveys of lands, obligations, and privileges undertaken by different Norman authorities. Unfortunately, no professional association undertook a census of physicians, nor did the royal government apparently consider such a count necessary.

Lost records inhibit any exhaustive modern tabulation, but national reports, local inquests, and property deeds occasionally name a healer as subject, beneficiary, or signatory witness. Such documentary appearances are quite rare for individuals who were presumably upstanding community leaders. Chronicle accounts feature physicians even less frequently. Nevertheless, there is no point in belaboring difficulties. The lack of complete evidence and the controversial nature of what does exist are well known. Less appreciated is how much can actually yet be discovered.

At least one contemporary bench-mark suggests the pervasive, still undetected strength of medical men in Anglo-Norman society. At some point in the second decade of the century an anonymous, unsophisticated clerk attempted the heroic task of codifying the laws of his country. Medicine has little place in his awkward summary, usually called the *Leges Henrici*, but his concluding section lists the monetary compensation for bodily injury and willful assault. In two instances the stipulated awards are based upon the assumption that medical attention will be readily available to victims. If this assessment is at all justified, it bespeaks a far larger health corps than one might at first expect.[1]

Further research confirms the law clerk's optimism by uncovering a surprising number of physicians.

Period	*Identifiable Practitioners*
400–1066	8
1066–1100	11
1100–1154	90

This accounting is much larger than any other total suggested for the Anglo-Norman era, but it is still only a fraction of the true unrecoverable figure.

Happily, these new statistics can be given a certain measure of life. First, a roster of the names, dates, and locations of the individual practitioners is in order. Until new evidence appears, this listing must demonstrate the strength and vitality of Anglo-Norman practitioners. In order to encourage detailed reference and to eliminate repetitive citations, the specific documentation for each healer has been cataloged alphabetically in Appendix 1 at the end of this book.

From the six and a half centuries between the departure of the Romans

Table 1. Roster of Physicians from 500 to 1154

Physician	Status	Location	Date
500–1066			
1. Melus	?	Lelyn Peninsula	c.500
2. Cynefrid	layman	Ely	679–695
3. Bald	?	?	900/50
4. Cild	?	?	900/50
5. Dun	?	?	900/50
6. Oxa	?	?	900/50
7. Baldwin*	monk/abbot	Bury	1059–1097
8. Master Adelard*	canon	Waltham	1060–1108
1066–1100			
1. Master Adelard*	canon	Waltham	1060–1108
2. Albert of Bec	monk	Canterbury	c. 1070
3. Aluricus	monk	Winchester	c. 1087
4. Argentien	layman	Ely	1066
5. Baldwin*	monk/abbot	Bury	1059–1097
6. Eudo	monk	Winchester	late 11th cent.
7. Faritius*	monk	Malmesbury	1078–1117
8. John*	cleric/bishop	Bath	1088–1122
9. Maurice	monk	Canterbury	1070
10. Nigel*	layman	many shires	1086–1107/28
11. Theobald	layman (?)	Devon	1086
12. Gilbert Maminot**	cleric/bishop	Lisieux	1066–1101
13. Goisbertus**	monk	Saint Evroult	1078/83
1100–1154			
1. Master Adam	layman	York	c. 1150
2. Master Adelard*	canon	Waltham	1060–1108
3. Ailred	monk/abbot	Rievaulx	1110–1167
4. Andrew	monk (?)	Rochester	1108
5. Arnold	layman	Suffolk	1133/43–1153/64
6. Baldwin	layman (?)	Essex	1138/48
7. Bernard	layman	York/Durham	1143/49–1142/54
8. Bertram	layman (?)	London	1132/54
9. Clarembald	priest	Exeter/London	1107–1133
10. Edward	layman	Totnes	c. 1140
11. Master Ernulf	?	Ely	1133/45–1162/69
12. Ernulf	layman (?)	London	1040/44
13. Faritius*	abbot	Abingdon	1078–1117
14. Geoffrey	?	Abingdon (?)	1108
15. Geoffrey	layman (?)	Norfolk	c. 1150
16. Gervase	layman	Durham	1124/53–1156/74
17. Gilbert	layman	London	1128/38
18. Master Gilbert	monk (?)	Peterborough	c. 1130
19. Gilbert of Falaise	layman	Nottingham	1130
20. Gregory	monk	Malmesbury	–1106

*multiple listing
**visitor to England, not a resident

Table 1.   Roster of Physicians from 500 to 1154 (Continued)

Physicians	Status	Location	Date
21. Gregory	cleric	Warwick	1115/19
22. Gregory	layman	Staffordshire	1127/38
23. Grimbald	layman	many shires	1101–1138
24. Master Guy	canon	Merton	1114–1124
25. Haldane	layman (?)	Lincoln	c. 1140
26. Henry	layman (?)	York	1147/53–1150/59
27. M. Henry of Bolwick	layman (?)	Norfolk	1153/68–1190/1203
28. Master Herbert	?	Durham	–1153
29. Hugh	monk/abbot	Chertsey	1107–1128
30. Master Hugh	?	Kenilworth	c. 1130
31. Hu[gh]	?	Essex	1123/33–1141/54
32. Hugh	cleric	Totnes	c. 1130
33. Hugh	?	Lewes	c. 1140
34. Hugh	layman (?)	York	1142/55–1154/81
35. Hugh	cleric (?)	Norfolk	c. 1150
36. Humphrey	layman	Hertford	c. 1150
37. Iwod	layman (?)	London	1140/44
38. Jocelin	?	Chichester	1147/63–1154/63
39. John*	cleric/bishop	Bath	1088–1122
40. John	layman (?)	London	1128/38
41. John	cleric	Totnes	c. 1130
42. John	monk	Ely	1133/69–1162/69
43. John	?	Essex	c. 1140–1171
44. Master John	?	Lincoln	1140/76–1150/95
45. John	?	York	1150/70
46. Lambert	cleric	Yorkshire	1135/41–1165/77
47. Lucian	?	Essex	1120/1140
48. Mark	cleric	?	–1124
49. Melbethe	layman	Cumberland	–1126
50. Miles	?	Northampton	1136/41
51. Nigel*	layman	many shires	1086–1107/28
52. Nigel of Calne	cleric	London/Sarum	1107/12–1130
53. Osmar	layman (?)	Middlesex	1150/52
54. Pain	?	Winchester	1148
55. Paulinus	layman (?)	York	1122/33–1166/81
56. Pedro Alfonso	layman	Gloucester	1062–1142
57. Peter	cleric	Bedford	1136/38
58. Peter de Quincy	monk	Yorkshire	1140–1156
59. Peter	layman (?)	Canterbury	c. 1143
60. Peter	cleric	Leicester	c. 1153
61. Picot	cleric	Gloucester	1147–1166/83
62. Rainier	layman	Abingdon	–1117
63. Ralph	cleric (?)	Exeter	1107/37
64. Ralph	layman	Lincoln	–1130
65. Ralph	monk (?)	St. Albans	1119/46
66. Master Ralph	cleric (?)	Lincoln	1148/66–1170
67. Ramelmus	monk	Much Wenlock	1101
68. Ranulf	cleric/monk	Montacute	–1120

Table 1. Roster of Physicians from 500 to 1154 (Continued)

Physicians	Status	Location	Date
69. Richard	?	Winchester	1148–1185
70. Robert	?	Warwick (?)	1119/53
71. Robert	?	Oxford	1136/38
72. Robert	layman	Yorkshire	1130/60
73. Robert	layman	York	1143/77
74. Roger	canon (?)	Lincoln	1151
75. M. Roger of Glou- cester	layman (?)	Gloucester	1148/63
76. Roland	?	Canterbury	1120/22
77. M. Serlo of Arundel	cleric	Arundel	1136–1160
78. Master Stephen	layman	Leicester	1148/57
79. Walter	cleric	Kenilworth	1136/43
80. Master Walter	?	York	1137/40
81. Master Walter	?	Norfolk	c. 1140
82. Walter	layman (?)	Lewes	1146/54
83. M. Walter Daniel	monk	Rievaulx	1125–1167
85. William	layman	Lincoln	1114
86. William	layman (?)	Bedford	–1124
87. William	layman (?)	Revesby	1142/43
87. William	?	Winchester	1148
88. Master William	cleric (?)	Canterbury	1148/54
89. William	canon	London	1149/57
90. Wulfric	priest/hermit	Somerset	c. 1080–1154

and the arrival of the Normans, only eight physicians can be identified by name. Melus was certainly British or Roman, not Saxon, and he must have been one of the last to retain any vestige of the classical medical tradition. Cynefrid seems to have been a layman, who ministered to the religious at Ely for more than sixteen years. Cild, Dun, and Oxa are mentioned in *Bald's Leechbook*, and Adelard and Baldwin were foreigners who came to England in the very last years of the Confessor. The complex medical literature of the Saxons indicates that there must have been a host of other practitioners. Every so often a fleeting glimpse of one of these lost professionals is unexpectedly revealed. For example, the existence of a highly skilled surgeon who successfully performed trephinations on half a dozen patients in East Anglia in the late sixth century has recently been detected. He must have had many colleagues.[2]

In any event, the number of Saxon doctors seems insignificant beside the Conquest register, a list overwhelmed by the host of early twelfth-century practitioners. Yet here, too, there are many additional but unidentifiable physicians. The records continually speak of people consulting doctors, but leave them unnamed. For example, Bishop John of Rochester (1125–37) visited several anonymous physicians about his severe eye troubles, and there are references to an earlier physician in Bishop Gundulph's time (1077–1108). In fact, it has been calculated that at least ten percent of the English pilgrims who were recorded as receiving cures at major pilgrimage shrines had previously sought medical assistance.[3]

Doctors renowned for their sanctity or their royal connections have left the best traces. The court physicians will be examined shortly, but their colleagues are not complete ciphers, and much can be said about their common characteristics. Although no single entry can generate a full-scale biographical portrait, a composite of all the doctors' careers does enlarge our view of Anglo-Norman society.[4]

Finding the medieval physicians can be quite challenging. The professional title universally employed in the early twelfth century was *medicus*. Oddly enough, many practitioners did not feel it desirable to use such a signature, or to use it consistently. The motives for such reticence are unclear, but they effectively hide the status of unknown numbers of physicians. A healer sometimes signed different charters in different ways, using a title one moment and none the next. Occasionally his designation even varied within the same document.

The term medicus was highly complimentary, but not absolutely precise. Frequently it seemed to applaud an individual's curative skill rather than to denote his formal training or daily occupation. God was often invoked as the Great Physician or the Physician of All Men's Souls. Earthly healers were also saluted in a kind of prayer. For example, in 1092, when Earl Hugh of Chester wrote from his sickbed to Anselm, then abbot of Bec, he called him a physician and begged him to come to England and heal him. Despite his illness, the baron clearly intended his words to be a flattering tribute, not a medical title.[5]

The distinction was often more obscure. Master Guy, a famous Italian teacher, became an Austin canon at Merton Priory in 1114. Although unsuccessful in administration at Merton's daughter-houses in Taunton and Bodmin, Guy was an admired spiritual counselor who, according to Rainald of Merton, also cured bodily ailments as, or just as, an expert physician (*unde velut peritus medicus*) would. Similarly, Ailred of Rievaulx visited and healed the sick; when his biographer called him a medicus, the intended meaning was again a bit ambiguous.

A few instances of such debatable terminology notwithstanding, a good rule of thumb is to consider a man a physician if he was called a medicus or said to be expert in the art of medicine. Obvious cases of hyperbole, like that of Anselm, can easily be discounted. There is no early indication of specialization, but after mid-century, the old and somewhat more elegant words, *physicus* and *cirurgicus*, would again become common. Some scholars have described Henrican doctors by the ancient Saxon title *leech*. This seems reasonable, and it was probably used at the time. However it has not yet been found accompanying any personal name in the Norman period. *Leech* did become a family patronymic, and it is theoretically conceivable that *medicus* was sometimes intended as a surname rather than a professional designation. Occupational cognomens like *miller, smith,* and *cook* quickly became family names; but there is no evidence for this happening to *medicus,* and many *medici* can definitely be observed practicing medicine.[6]

John, the physician of Essex, presents a revealing example of the variant uses of medical terminology. All references to him fall between 1156 and 1171, but granted the long careers of most doctors, he undoubtedly practiced under Stephen and probably under Henry I. When he died, evidently in August, 1171, John was receiving a royal honorarium of a penny a day. This modest sum was a rather traditional expression of the royal bounty; it was the standard wage for a common soldier, the daily dole for a blind man, and the stipend of an inmate at several royal hospitals. There was nothing generous about John's retainer, but it may have been a type of pension, the first regular medical perquisite known. He had been receiving the same rate every year since at least 1156. His title changed over the years, however. In the third year of Henry II's reign the physician appeared in the pipe roll as John *minutori.* This rather rare word meant phlebotomist, or bloodletter. For the next two years he was called John *medicus.* In 1160 and thereafter he was termed *dubbedent* and *adubedent* (or *addubendt*), unclear words that may have meant dentist, the earliest so mentioned.

The only other instance of a person named phlebotomist is that of Wlmarus the minutor, a layman who attested a charter for Saint Paul's cathedral in 1138x1152.* The list of witnesses is very long and Wlmarus was placed among the laymen, fifty-sixth in a total of seventy-six men of London.[7] Since he was not described as a medicus, he was not listed in the roster of physicians, but, in view of John the minutor's later identification, perhaps phlebotomists should regularly be considered physicians. At about the same time as Wlmarus, a Hugh "cum dentibus" attests a charter.[8] Perhaps he was another dentist. There is also a lone reference to a possible veterinary surgeon. In 1109x1131 Bishop Hervey of Ely confirmed certain lands to Haldeyn the baker and referred to his practice of bleeding horses. Note that Haldane is also the name of a physician of this time.[9]

No female practitioners have yet come to light in Norman England. Naturally there must have been innumerable midwives, but they do not appear in the records. The absence of women physicians is more surprising than one might believe. In the late eleventh century a woman was said to be the most learned person at Salerno, and Dame Trotula, author of a famous book on gynecology, may well have been active then, too. A German nun, Hildegard of Bingen (1098–1179), was renowned for her medical researches, and a lady practitioner was known in France. Female healers appeared later in medieval Britain, but evidently not in King Henry's time.[10]

---

*The *x* signifies "between." (Read "sometime between 1138 and 1152".)

On the other hand, English women took a decisive, even commanding, role in encouraging hospital construction. They put in relatively few appearances in royal and ecclesiastical charters, but in private family deeds they are vigorously represented. Very often someone's wife, widow, or mother initiated a charitable gift. Sheer numbers were against them, however, for, in an unusual demographic imbalance, men both significantly outnumbered and outlived women.[11]

The physician's personal names are worth considering for a moment. They run from Adam to Wulfric, but display little imagination and merely reflect the common range of most Anglo-Norman Christian names. Fifty different given names are represented on the physicians' roster, but Hugh, John, Peter, Walter, and William were favorites. Conceivably a few multiple listings might denote one doctor in two locations rather than separate men of the same name, but the circumstances of the different occurrences invariably argue for distinct individuals. One might have expected to encounter other names, such as James, Michael, or Nicholas, some of the age's most popular saints; or Bartholomew, Giles, and Leonard, familiar patron saints of hospitals and certain diseases. There were no surnames, although these were just coming into fashion. However, Gilbert of Falaise, Henry of Bolwick, Nigel of Calne, Peter of Quincy, Roger of Gloucester, Serlo of Arundel, and John and Walter of York coupled their personal names with a place in a manner that was quite common at the time.

Most of the names are unmistakably Norman. Does this mean that most physicians came from that conquering race rather than from the subject people? The extensive native medical literature and the fact that only about ten thousand Normans lived in a total population of about two million indicate that most practitioners ought to have been Saxons. In the above list, however, only Ailred and Wulfric are definitely Saxon names. Edward and Paulinus suggest an English heritage, and the names Haldane, Melbethe, and Osmar reflect Scandinavian descent, another important strain in the host population.

Most documents involve Norman affairs, so this phenomenon may be a case of like treating like. Moreover, the conquerors were quite adept at obliterating the contributions of their defeated foes, even a generation after Hastings. Then too, some Saxons and Danes changed their names to conform to the new order, just as Queen Matilda abandoned her given name, Edith. This was especially true for clerics, many of whom changed their names anyway when entering religious life. For example, Bartholomew (c. 1120–93), the hermit of Farne, near Durham, was first called Tostig, but when that met with local ridicule, he began to call himself William. After becoming a monk he adopted the name Bartholomew. Such alteration was probably fairly common, but it rarely appears in the records. A rather poignant example comes from a gravestone at Saint Augustine's monastery in

Canterbury, where an early monk had his two names inscribed, "Edzie son of Edward who was also called Gerald." Later, in the same town, Archbishop William Corbeil decided he disliked the name of one of his associates, Siward, so he took to calling him Simon. Another Saxon took the very explicit name Norman. Change did not always lead to favor. There was one monk at Bury, with the distinctly un-English name of Baldwin, who was elected abbot in 1107, but the king prevented his installation because the monk was a Saxon.[12]

Thus, the list of physicians may well include several other Saxons who are disguised by their Norman-sounding names. Nevertheless, the suspicion still persists that after 1066 more Normans than Saxons were active in medicine. Indeed, the increasing knowledge of the personalities of post-Conquest physicians must be occasioned, in part at least, by their own rising prestige and changing social status. It is a curious peculiarity of England, however, that physicians there never attained the special dignity of their colleagues elsewhere in the British Isles. Ireland had long honored savants of all kinds, and tenth-century Welsh laws reserved high places in the palace for physicians, offering them fixed salaries. Some of this deference continued right through the twelfth century. It is hardly surprising, therefore, that Irish and Welsh practitioners felt no need to move to England.[13]

Although a good number of early Anglo-Norman physicians had been born in foreign lands, this tendency decreased in time. Faritius, Guy, and Grimbald were Italians. Master Adelard was from Flanders, John of Bath from Tours, Peter de Quincy from France, and Pedro Alfonso was a converted Spanish Jew. A number of physicians were born in Normandy, but more were sons of immigrants.

No specifics have survived about the training and education of Henrican physicians. Presumably those raised in Italy had some likelihood of attending classes at Salerno or at Monte Cassino, the mother abbey that sheltered Constantine the African. As time went on, more and more English sought foreign training. The results did not please all observers. In 1159, the classical enthusiast, John of Salisbury, issued a long complaint about many of his contemporaries; he was especially critical of medical students. His caustic humor is worth quoting at length.

Others, becoming cognizant of their inadequate grounding in philosophy, have departed to Salerno or to Montpellier, where they have become medical students. Then suddenly, in the twinkling of an eye, they have blossomed forth as the same kind of physicians that they had previously been philosophers. Stocked with fallacious empirical rules [for handling various cases] they return after a brief interval to practice with sedulity what they have learned. Ostentatiously they quote Hippocrates and Galen, pronounce mysterious words, and have [their] aphorisms ready to apply to all cases. Their strange terms serve as thunderbolts which stun the minds of their fellow men. They are revered as omnipotent, because that is what they boast and promise.

However, I have observed that there are two rules which they are more especially prone to recall and put into practice. The first is from Hippocrates (whom they misinterpret): "Where there is indigence, one ought not to labor." Verily they have judged it unfitting, and foreign to their profession, to attend the needy and those who are either loath or unable to pay the full price, if it be only for their words. Their second maxim does not come, as I recollect, from Hippocrates, but has been added by enterprising doctors: "Take [your fee] while the patient is in pain." When a sick person is tortured by suffering, it is a particularly auspicious time for demanding one's price. For then the anguish of the illness and the avarice of the one affecting to cure it collaborate. If the patient recovers, the credit will go to the doctor, whereas it he grows worse, the medico's reputation will still be enhanced, since he has already predicted such an outcome to his intimates. The wily physician has, indeed, made it impossible for his predictions not to be realized. To one he has foretold that the patient's health will be restored; while to another he has declared that it is impossible for the sick man to recover. If a patient has the good fortune to survive, he does so easily, except so far as the bungling medico may delay his recovery. But if he is fated to succumb, then, as Solinus Sidonius remarks, "he is killed with full rites."[14]

Obviously, John of Salisbury was an unfriendly witness. In fact, he was a small frail man who always had unpleasant experiences with physicians and his jaundiced views should be taken with a grain of salt. Although his unique satire is unsupported by other contemporary testimony, it does reveal another side of twelfth-century medicine. A few Englishmen can be identified at Salerno about this period, including the two Cambridgeshire brothers, Matthew and Warin (d. 1195), who later became monks at Saint Albans. One wonders if they were part of the company John ridiculed.

Medical study was a never-ending process. Some Henrican physicians traveled widely in their later years and undoubtedly examined continental facilities and techniques. Hugh of Chertsey, for example, went to Rome in 1116. Two of his traveling companions fell ill on the road, but his medical skill did not initially help them very much. Another practitioner, Grimbald, the royal physician, followed the king to the continent several times, as did Nigel of Calne. Master Herbert of Durham kept his medical library up to date with all the latest translations.

A hazy reflection of English interest in scholastic medicine can be discerned in the unfounded rumors that Oxford and Cambridge each housed a medical school in the early twelfth century. The Oxford school, for which there is no valid contemporary evidence whatsoever, was supposedly established by Jewish physicians. The instructional record at Cambridge is not much more secure. One writer of dubious veracity would have readers believe that five monks from the abbey of Saint Evroult in Normandy set up a school at Cottenham near Cambridge. Their leader, Geoffrey, who later served as abbot of Crowland from 1109 to 1124, supposedly taught medicine. If this questionable account has any value, Geoffrey, who is not in the above register, should probably be considered a physician himself. There

were important hospitals in the two towns and some sort of casual instruction may have been offered there, but nothing of greater, or at least enduring, significance seems possible.[15] On the other hand, it is worth
remembering that Warin and Matthew, sons of a modest Cambridge family,
went to Salerno, and that Adam, from nearby Balsham, was highly educated
and already a famous philosopher by 1132.

About 20 percent of the practitioners called themselves master (*magister*).
Whatever distinction this title conferred, its nature is obscure now. Some
modern scholars claim the title meant that the individual was in minor
orders, that he was a university graduate, or that he was a teacher in the
schools. While partly true, these definitions are too facile for general application in Norman times. Dozens and dozens of men—even cooks, masons,
and ironsmiths, as well as teachers and chaplains—adopted the usage. The
phrase did not merely occur as "master cook," either, but rather as "Master
Robert the ironsmith."[16]

Of even greater interest, some physicians, like Serlo of Arundel, preferred
the title of magister to that of medicus. In one of the many cases where two
physicians were found together, there appears the unusual joint attestation,
"Master Ernulf and Iwod the physicians." Unless this is a scribal error, some
meaningful, almost condescending, distinction was intended. The actual
word *doctor* was also used, but apparently more as an academic than a medical title.[17]

The title *master* somehow involved education and recognition, but real
status was determined by whether a man was a layman, a secular clergyman,
a regular canon, or a monk. Separating the clergy from the laity would later
become easy: if a physician had children, he fell among the laity. The early
twelfth century was a period of transition, however, and the church's widely
promulgated program of reform, which included mandatory celibacy, was
slow to take hold in Britain. The married clergy, particularly the rural clergy,
were not only reluctant to leave their own wives but also unwilling to let the
tradition of clerical marriage die at all. Thus several generations of twelfth-
century clerks can be traced. Bishops rarely fathered children after consecration, but Ralph of Orkney, who never visited his distant diocese but
regularly officiated in his native Yorkshire, was known to have had several
children. At least one of his sons, Paulinus, became a cleric, the master of
the great hospital of Saint Peter in York. He, too, had children of his own.[18]
Thus the simple fact that a physician had heirs does not automatically indicate that he deserves lay status. On the other hand, if this condition is combined with a relatively low ranking in a series of charter witnesses—the
clergy were usually listed first—chances are good that the individual was a
layman. Fortunately, lay, clerical, and monastic states were often more explicitly announced.

The ninety practitioners can be divided in the following manner.

	Probable	Possible	Total	Percentage
Monks	8	4	12	13.3%
Austin canons	1	—	1	1.1%
Other clergy	18	4	22	24.4%
Laymen	22	13	35	38.8%
Unclear	20	—	20	22.2%

Thus, considerably more than a third of the known physicians appear to have been laymen. This statistical proportion, probably much greater in reality, highlights an accelerating twelfth-century trend as medicine increasingly passed from the domain of clerical control to become a lay and learned specialty. The reformed papacy enthusiastically supported this movement by condemning any monastic practice of medicine that involved financial profits. Some of the practitioners must have sensed that the tide was with the laity or that most people would assume that physicians were laymen. Therefore, in attesting documents they carefully identified themselves as *clericus et medicus*. Clarembald, Lambert, and Walter used this emphatic formula.

The social background of physicians does not stand out clearly in the records. Those who were monks presumably came from the same class of wholly free landowners as did most of their brethern. Certainly, Ailred and Wulfric had parents of comfortable, but not luxurious, means. Most physicians who were secular clerics or laymen probably shared the same heritage. Other practitioners came from different social strata. For example, Richard of Sunderland was a man of lowly birth, a bound laborer who cut thatch as part of his work. His whole family was evidently quite pious. Richard reportedly had a vision of three green men who tempted him to sin and then struck him dumb when he refused their blandishments. He was later restored to speech through the intercession of Saint Cuthbert. His nephew was miraculously cured of a deformed foot by the same saint. Richard's unnamed father was once laid up with an illness he had healed in others but could not overcome in himself. He therefore resorted to a familiar devotional practice, taking his own measurements with a rope and offering a wax candle of the same total length to Saint Cuthbert's shrine. Only then was he cured. The chronicler said this was a lesson to demonstrate that healing was a gift of God, not man.

Richard's father was probably of the same low social status as his son. Although the father was not called a medicus, he clearly treated many sufferers in his locale. He may have been a physician, but more likely he was one of the many exponents of folk or paraprofessional medicine. Later in the century another Yorkshireman was clearly both a medicus and a serf.[19]

Few family teams of physicians have yet come to light. By mid-century a father-son pair, Peter and John, were known at Canterbury, and shortly thereafter the Jews of London could boast a similar combination. Later the monks of Saint Albans numbered among their members the brother doctors Matthew and Warin.

Physicians were respected professionals, but early twelfth-century society did not defer to them. It has already been noted that healers occasionally neglected to record their medical proficiency or disguised it under the more inclusive term *master*. Other healers stressed a clerical as well as a medical status. Naturally, physicians who became bishops and abbots dropped their medical designation altogether, even when they kept up their practice. Physicians who did indicate their profession only attained a middling rank in charter attestations. In absolute numbers and relative placement they fell well behind the clerks, chaplains, and knights, but they also trailed the proud cooks, who witnessed innumerable charters, and the industrious secretaries, who self-consciously recorded their own names and occupation. Physicians were about even with engineers, carpenters, and masons in the frequency and precedence of their appearances.

Niceties of form and title ought not be exaggerated. For all its emphasis on such matters, the early twelfth century was remarkably fluid in its classifications. Even the eight physicians who directly served the royal court were rather casual about their status. Only two of them, Clarembald and Ranulf, ever called themselves physicians of the king, and none of them used the antiquated title *archiater*, personal attendant to a king.[20]

Several physicians were known to be in actual medical practice: Ailred, Faritius, Grimbald, Gregory of Malmesbury, Hugh, Peter de Quincy, Ramelmus, Robert of Yorkshire, Walter Daniel, Wulfric of Haselbury, and probably Gervase of Durham. The brief references to them are not always flattering. The three monks, Gregory, Hugh, and Ramelmus, were mentioned because of their inability to cure certain patients. On the other hand, Robert of York, an obscure local doctor, was rewarded by a grateful patient whom he had helped. Peter de Quincy, an impetuous, headstrong monk, braved his way into prison to treat his feudal lord and was later rewarded with enough property to build a new abbey.

Some of the most detailed, but least complimentary, remarks concern anonymous physicians. William of Malmesbury rather maliciously reported two instances. When Hugh of Orival, Bishop of London from 1075 to 1085, contracted leprosy doctors advised him to be castrated. The operation healed nothing and only increased his shame. On the other hand, his successor, Maurice of London (1086–1107), was supposedly urged by physicians to "provide for the health of his body by the dispersal of his humours." After this oblique phrasing the monk added his own unambiguous evaluation of this rationale for incontinence: "Unhappy indeed is the man who protects the state of his flesh at the risk of his soul."[21]

According to two other gossipy chroniclers, William of Newburgh and Roger of Howden, writing eight decades after the event, when Archbishop

Thomas of York lay dying in 1114 he was told by his doctor that intercourse with a woman was the only remedy for his illness. Some advisers urged him to accept this guidance, claiming that God would not be offended since the act would be done solely for medical reasons and not for carnal lust. Surprisingly, the prelate supposedly agreed. A beautiful woman was brought to his room. Later, however, when the doctor inspected the archbishop's urine it was revealed that Thomas had only feigned acceptance in order to placate his friends. These men then strongly rebuked the patient, who finally reasserted his principles and declared that he was not going to lose the immortal glory of chastity for the sake of his mortal flesh. "Shame," he thundered, "upon a malady which requires sensuality for its cure." Perhaps he would have done better to castigate his entire entourage rather than his own condition. The pure man tempted by a lovely seductress conveniently placed in his bedroom is an old theme, and the tales doubtless had a didactic purpose, but they cannot be accepted as reliable accounts of Anglo-Norman medical practice.[22]

Deathbed sex evidently fascinated some clerical historians. In 1119 Baldwin, the count of Flanders, attacked Arques. Amidst the thick of battle his helmit was battered with repeated blows and he evidently sustained an injury to the brain. William of Malmesbury reported that men said — note the attribution to rumor once more — that Baldwin's disorder increased because he had eaten garlic and goose early in the day and would not abstain from carnal intercourse at night. King Henry even sent over a skilled but unnamed physician, but to no avail. This, by the way, is the sole reference to military medicine in Henry's reign. The particular physician was most likely directly attached to the king, however, rather than assigned to the army. Perhaps it was Grimbald who normally accompanied him, or Hugh of Chertsey or Nigel of Calne, who were both in France at the time.[23]

Among the identifiable practices, that of Ramelmus is especially interesting for several reasons: his activity can be pinpointed precisely; he can be seen treating the poor rather than the rich, who usually figure so prominently in documents; and he was probably typical of a whole class of unrecorded physicians. Such men would inevitably have considered the welfare of brother religious their primary responsibility, but they would also willingly treat external patients. Ramelmus's monastery, Much Wenlock in Shropshire (where one can still see the twelfth-century infirmary), was an ancient Saxon nunnery refounded for men about 1079 by Robert of Montgomery, earl of Shrewsbury. It was a fairly large Cluniac priory dedicated to Saint Michael and to Saint Milburga (d. 715), a princess whose relics, rediscovered in 1100, produced several miracles for the local populace. These wonders were investigated within the year by a cardinal legate who wrote a report of his visit after his return to Rome.

Ramelus was accustomed to treating people from all the nearby villages and to supplying them regularly with needed medicines. He was unable to cure one woman, but through the intervention of Saint Milburga she eventually vomited forth a great worm. Her husband later encased it in a special wooden box and brought it to the church. The sainted Saxon princess seems to have particularly attracted women and children to her care and to have been expecially helpful to people afflicted with blindness and leprosy.

When one peasant's son was miraculously restored to sight, an interesting test of the wonder's authenticity was recorded. The monks carefully observed how the boy's first sighted identification of objects depended upon his former tactile interpretation of their shape and materials. Such examinations were not uncommon when miracles were reported.[24] The cure of a poor girl reveals something about how rural people handled their own problems. The twelve-year-old daughter of a leper who had died from his disease also contracted the malady, but she was still cared for at home by her mother and stepfather until healed by holy Milburga. In another case an outspoken woman annoyed the compiler of these miracles by complaining that saints rarely cured lepers. Ramelmus's unspectacular services may seem lost amidst the saint's miracles, but this is to misread the account. Evidently most people regularly consulted him, and only incurable patients turned to Milburga.

Ramelmus's solitary fight against illness was blessed by the patron of his monastery. Other physicians invoked the saints, too, but they also frequently consulted one another. One of the amazing aspects of the twelfth century is the continual discovery of extensive contacts among people. In his isolated part of the world, Ramelmus helped entertain a Roman cardinal, one of the first to visit Britain. More to the point of this investigation, at least fifteen of these physicians knew one or more of their fellow doctors, despite the hazards of travel and the necessarily local orientation to life. Moreover, there were numerous conferences of other unnamed practitioners.[25]

How long did such men serve? The available data is rather thin, but some examples are suggestive. Ailred lived for fifty-seven years, but he was sick during much of his later life. Wulfric died at about age sixty-four, and Pedro Alfonso seems to have continued past eighty-four. Many of the listed physicians can be observed with careers of more than thirty years, and these are only partial segments. This length should not be surprising, and I emphasize it only because there still persists a mistaken view that most medieval people died young. A study of the lifespans of monks, many of whom survived into their eighties, would immediately contradict this impression. The average age of abbots who became saints was approximately seventy.[26] Many archdeacons, abbots, and even a few bishops had careers of forty years and more, not counting their earlier nonexecutive periods. Lay careers are notoriously more difficult to measure, but the lay physicians provide an interesting countrywide cross section. Assuming that doctors began to practice at about age twenty, most of them enjoyed a lifespan that stretched well into their sixth decade and beyond.

As befitted their professional interests and advanced training of whatever type, most physicians were bookish men—even the hermit, Wulfric, maintained a personal library. Ailred, Clarembald, Faritius, Pedro, Walter Daniel, and perhaps Gervase, were authors. Others, like Herbert and Ralph, were collectors. Their private preoccupation reflects the national trend of increasing book transcription. Moreover, when these practitioners do appear in the records, particularly as charter witnesses, they are often found associating with other learned men, especially local schoolmasters. It may seem unnecessary to stress such minor connections, but since twelfth-century doctors have rarely been credited with any intellectual interests it is well to redress the balance whenever possible. On the whole, the depth of their genuine scholarly concern probably varied as much as that of practitioners in any age.

One physician was a particularly avid bibliophile. Sometime before 1153 Master Herbert gave the monks of Durham a total of twenty-six different books, mostly classical medical texts. Shortly thereafter, certainly before 1163, a catalog was made of the Durham Cathedral library listing its holdings by donors' names. Herbert's collective gift and its constituent titles were thereby recorded. His twenty-six tracts of varying lengths were bound, apparently in Herbert's lifetime, into five or more volumes. Happily, two of these compendia still exist.[27]

One set of six treatises obtained by Doctor Herbert was sewn together and then bound between boards covered with white skin and fastened with a strap and pin. A prominent note atop the second page indicates that this collection was the gift of Master Herbert the physician.[28] The treatises are the same as those the Durham cataloger reported as being together in one volume, but the order is different and one number has disappeared. Later catalog descriptions and holes along the pages' outside margin indicate that the set was rearranged more than once. The works are in several different twelfth-century hands, which suggests that Herbert purchased them individually or had them copied at different places or by different men rather than commissioning them from one scribe. Six more of Herbert's treatises in another set were also reproduced by several copyists, some of whom used a rather small script and, as in the other volume, red and green initials.[29]

To judge from the full twenty-six titles, Herbert conscientiously tried to keep abreast of all the latest technical literature, especially the Moslem versions of Greek, Roman, and Jewish medical classics, which had been appearing in Latin translations since about 1077. At Salerno and Monte Cassino, fired by the zeal of his recent conversion, Constantine worked unceasingly to prepare such translations. His thirty-seven various editions soon became the backbone of the Salernitan curriculum, and scribes could not keep up with the demand for texts.

Most of Herbert's titles had first become available through Constantine's adaptations, and the Durham physician acquired some of the best parts of the total corpus. Perhaps this reflects some personal experience with the school of Salerno. Certainly students there were simultaneously taking notes on the very same authors that Herbert purchased. Moreover, his selections continued to be required university reading and served as authoritative clinical reference books for centuries. A syllabus for students at Montpellier in 1309, for example, almost mirrors Herbert's own collection.[30]

All practitioners certainly did not possess the Durham master's extensive library, but many would have been familiar with the titles he selected. Herbert owned both practical manuals and theoretical tracts—general works of diagnosis, recipes for dyeing the hair, alphabetically arranged prescriptions, detailed surgical handbooks, and even a discussion of mental illness. There were two herbals, two collections of simple drugs, two treatises on urine, and a lapidary. Fever was considered an illness rather than a sympton and received individual attention, as did epidemics. Works by Hippocrates, Galen, Dioscorides, and Isaac Judaeus were there, but so were newer studies by contemporary authors like Master Roger of Salerno, Master Reginald of Montpellier, John Platerarius of Salerno, Constantine the African, and even the Waltham canon, Philip of Thaon.[31]

Many physicians would have been familiar with a shortened version of Dioscorides' herbal containing descriptions of seventy-one drugs. This Greek doctor once served in Nero's imperial army and some editions of his complete *materia medica* cataloged almost one thousand drugs. Sources included animal and mineral as well as vegetable substances. Master Herbert's more standard intermediate version listed about seven hundred entries. Even so, it was not an exact copy of an ancient exemplar, for the unknown twelfth-century editor replaced about fifteen of Dioscorides' descriptions with corresponding choices from another classical source fairly popular in Saxon England, the medical lapidary ascribed to a first-century Alexandrian magician, Daimegiron.[32]

Although alphabetized and written in a large, clear hand, Herbert's copy of the herbal may actually have been less functional than the shorter version. It lacked illustrations and probably exhausted anyone trying to master it. In a full lifetime an average physician could never encounter all the specimens listed. A few readers, perhaps even Herbert himself, made notes in the wide margins. Although this practice suggests careful use, the readers' industry evidently flagged after several dozen *A* descriptions, and entries under later letters received considerably less attention.

The short eleven-page alphabetical lapidary that Herbert ordered was evidently a work of Philip of Thaon. Although more naturalistic than the allegorical lapidary Philip made for Queen Adeliza, it, too, was written in Anglo-Norman verse. This use of the vernacular suggests that Herbert was of Norman descent or at least fluent in languages. There was not much magical, astronomical, or astrological writing in Herbert's personal library, but he did invest in at least one section of a famous semioccult tract, the

Secret of Secrets. Legend had it that Aristotle drafted this compendium of varied advice for his star pupil, Alexander the Great. Like many ancient texts it was preserved in an Arabic edition and eventually retranslated into Latin. Shortly before 1130 John of Seville published its medical portion, about 188 lines. The full work would have a great and complicated future and would also be used by Herbert's contemporary, Pedro Alfonso, the converted Spanish physician who served King Henry. John of Seville also translated Costa Ben Lucca's *Difference of Soul and Spirit*, a copy of which Herbert purchased.[33]

The Durham master also owned a little booklet composed by Pedro Alfonso. This double-column text was written in a clear, if rather cramped, hand, but the manuscript does not show much sign of use. It is filled with references to characters from Greece and Rome, such as Solon, Diogenes, Alexander, Caesar, and Cato the Elder. Although it unfortunately lacks the personal introductory remarks with which Pedro normally began his treatises, it was ascribed to him in the table of contents of the volume in which it was bound with several of Herbert's other books. Hardly one of the Spanish doctor's most interesting works, it was a rather uninspired selection on Herbert's part. However, his ownership of this and of the famed *Secret of Secrets*, which Pedro also knew, suggests some contact between the two physicians and perhaps a link with Spain as well as Salerno.[34]

There was also the interesting connection with Waltham. The bishop of Durham had controlled the Essex college for a generation after the Conquest, until Henry gave it to Matilda. Even after the separation, Waltham canons occasionally joined the Durham cathedral priory. Tall, good-looking, sweet-voiced Prior Lawrence of Durham (1149–54) had been a secular canon at Waltham Holy Cross before he came to Durham sometime before 1128. He was a poet who specialized in metrical composition and realistic descriptions of nature. It has been suggested that he may have personally drawn up the oldest catalog of Durham books, the list containing Herbert's gift. Richard, a former dean of Waltham, also retired to Durham. The two churches mirrored each other's architecture — although different in scale, both naves shared similar designs, including the striking, deeply carved chevrons on the columns. Master Adelard, the celebrated physician and educator of Waltham, was well known in the north, and later, the anniversary of his death was solemnly commemorated at Durham. Perhaps he inspired some of Herbert's choices, especially the purchase of one of Philip of Thaon's books.

The outreach of the Durham doctor was indeed impressive, but his interests did not always resemble those of other natural scientists. Theology and mathematics are not prominent in Herbert's collection, and only a few snippets of grammatical rules can be found. The familiar bestiary does not appear and miracle stories are absent; nor are there charms, incantations, or weird magical remedies. In fact, Herbert's selection shows a very evenhanded choice of useful works, like the surgical manuals and the herbals, and of theoretical studies, such as Constantine's translation of Haly Abbas's *Pantegni*. The latter book typifies the movement away from empirical analysis of concrete needs and toward the rarified speculations of academic medicine, a trend that would characterize the rest of the century's writing.

On the whole, Herbert's complete library seems to be the product of a quite secular, somewhat unimaginative, rather single-minded man. His costly expenditure of time and money bespeaks both a searching intellectual awareness and a lucrative professional practice. That an otherwise unknown physician in distant Durham would accumulate so much is one more indication of the responsible service of Henrican healers.

Herbert's books were not the only medical texts then collected in Durham. At least three other volumes of medical-calendrical-astronomical-etymological lore survive from the first half of the twelfth century. One is a masterpiece of calligraphy and has several interesting, if rather puzzling, drawings of untonsured physicians and chastely clad men preparing for cauterization.[35] Library catalogs indicate that there were once additional medical books in the cathedral, including one from, or by, a Gervase physicus. It is tempting to think this might be the known Gervase medicus of Durham.[36]

Herbert and Gervase were the most northerly practitioners in the long list, but there were physicians in all parts of the land. So far, they can be found in twenty-nine different shires. Important areas like Worcester and Hereford do not offer such evidence, but that is undoubtedly a result of the unevenness of the records. The concentration of nine men in London and Middlesex and twelve others in Yorkshire could be anticipated. What is strange is that Devon would support six doctors, three of whom were from the tiny town of Totnes.

The estimated population of the whole country at the time of the Domesday survey in 1086 has usually been placed at 1,500,000 souls, but it has become increasingly clear that this underrepresents large numbers of people, especially the richer, more independent peasants. A better guess for the early twelfth century would be the convenient round figure two million. Dividing this approximation by the total number of identified physicians produces a rather meaningless rate of one practitioner for every twelve thousand inhabitants. However, a more valid ratio of physicians to people can be obtained by measuring selected local areas. Totnes, for example, probably possessed only about six hundred individuals in 1100. If all three of its doctors were active at the same time and if they did not exclusively serve the gentry or the clergy, there was at least one physician available for every two hundred persons. Nearby Exeter, with an urban populace of around two thousand, would have a minimal ratio of one doctor for every one thousand citizens.[37]

When town and country names are similar it is difficult to determine

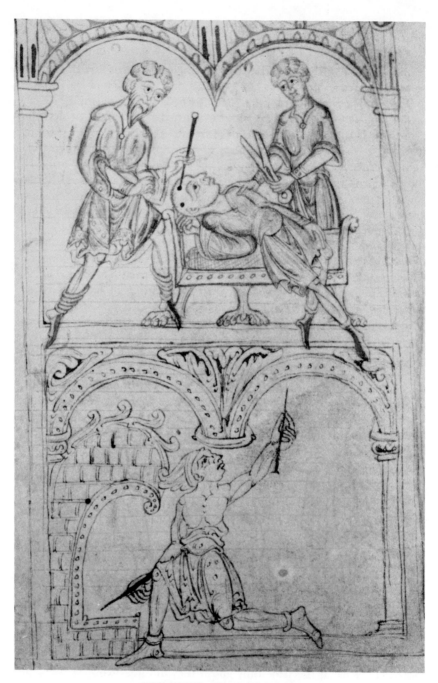

SURGERY IN DURHAM

The upper panel depicts a surgeon cauterizing the temples of a patient, who has just been shorn by the doctor's assistant. The lower register shows a strangely dressed associate heating the brands. Subsequent pages in the manuscript feature other physicians and partially dressed pa-

where a physician served. Most likely, he was active in both places, but centered in the town. Three examples are pertinent. Oxford town probably housed four thousand people in 1100. At least one physician, Robert, can be discovered working thereabout, although Geoffrey and Serlo also attested writs for local properties. Warwick, which had four resident practitioners was another active place. The town boasted about two hundred fifty houses for its fifteen hundred souls and even had a school, a mint, and a hospital, as had Oxford. The shire population may have reached seven thousand. York city suffered a decline under the rough times of early Norman rule, but it, too, was well endowed with health care facilities, especially the ancient hospital of Saint Peter. It also had more than twenty churches, which dispensed other charity. At the turn of the century the population may have been about five thousand, and several of the dozen shire doctors undoubtedly practiced in town. London, of course, was always a place unto itself, but if its populace numbered twenty thousand individuals, its medical ratio was not unlike that of other parts of the country.[38]

Winchester may offer the best model. In 1148 the bishop undertook a survey of all the urban property owners. Included were the names of three physicians. Mention was also made of the fact that Grimbald the doctor, had once owned land there, but he had died at least a decade earlier. Presuming the three practitioners to be residents and accepting the estimated population as eight thousand, it seems that Winchester maintained at least one doctor for every twenty-seven hundred city dwellers. Moreover, this would be a minimal estimate since the cathedral abbey usually had a physician among its members and other healers were undoubtedly attached to the great hospital of Saint Cross, just outside the town.[39]

Towns probably housed about 10 percent of the population. If seven of them can claim a ratio of roughly one physician for every two thousand people, and if this proportion was generally true of the whole country, England was very well served by its medical corps. Certainly there are parts of Britain and the United States which have even poorer ratios today; numerous parts of the world do not even approach it.

Furthermore, if this estimate holds up, it suggests that the full Anglo-Norman medical community would have boasted almost a thousand members. The ninety thus far identified therefore become a very respectable sample of the whole. It could also be argued that, since medieval medicine involved little specialization and less ongoing research, and since midwives handled most cases of childbirth, a desirable twelfth-century ratio of doctors

---

tients exhibiting their cautery scars. None of the physicians is tonsured. The scenes conclude a miscellaneous collection of medical and astrological treatises made in Durham about 1100x1128. By permission of the Dean and Chapter of Durham Cathedral, Ms. Hunter 100, fo. 119.

to population need not have been as low as it would be today. Significantly, no instance has come to light where a person complained that medical service was not available when needed.

A comparison with the medical contingent of other nations is also enlightening. France, a land with a far larger population and area, lists somewhat fewer physicians in the period 1100–54. There was also a smaller increase from the eleventh to the twelfth century. Several of the men counted were Norman residents whose ruler for most of the period was the king of England. Moreover, French healers were quite unevenly distributed throughout their country. A full 20 percent had connections with Chartres, and there were other very substantial groupings at Angers and at Marmoutier, near Tours.[40]

Like their English counterparts, the French monarchs associated with learned physicians, particularly those with pronounced astrological abilities, but the results were somewhat mixed. Whatever their own failings, none of England's physicians gained the ridicule that came to the French royal doctor whom people called John the Blockhead (*surdus*). Evidently he prescribed a potion for Henry I of France (d. 1060) but inadvertently neglected to watch the conditions under which the monarch took his medicine. The Capetian died soon afterward and John had to live with the shame for the rest of his life. (Actually, he was probably lucky to have outlived the incident at all.) A monk of Marmoutier, Ralph the ill-tonsured (*mala corona*, d. 1062), was another physician who reflects the continental trait of not taking doctors too seriously.[41]

Comparative statistics for other lands are even more difficult to obtain. Syria under Saladin presents an additional model from beyond Christendom. From his nineteen-year reign some twenty-three physicians are known, eleven of whose biographies were later recorded and eleven of whom were directly attached to Saladin's own service.[42]

A few English physicians deliberately emphasized a regional connection. Gilbert called himself the physician of Peterborough. Paulinus and Walter signed as physicians of York, and William identified himself as the physician of Bourne. Early in his career Lambert attested as medicus of Clitheroe. The usage implies service to a specific area rather than to an individual patron, but its significance ought not to be exaggerated. Physicians held themselves accountable to people, not to municipal systems. These men had definite local ties they thought worth proclaiming, but most loyalties were personal, and many of the listed physicians found powerful baronial protectors. King Henry was the premier medical patron, but his example was followed by many other lords.

The Beaumont family had a particular interest in health care. One of their doctors, Gregory, carried the feudal sense of identification further than anyone else by calling himself the physician of Henry, earl of Warwick.

Master Hugh and Walter also knew this lord, and Robert attended his son. Henry's brother, Robert de Beaumont, the count of Meulan and principal lay adviser to King Henry, considered himself an authority on nutrition as well as politics. After returning from the Holy Land he adopted the Byzantine routine of eating only one large meal a day. He attributed his robust health to the change and urged his associates to follow his lead.[43] Robert entrusted the education of his twin sons to the Italian physician, Abbot Faritius of Abingdon, who so often served the royal household. His confidence was not misplaced, for the boys quickly developed a reputation for learning and rhetoric. One of them, Robert II, earl of Leicester, employed a physician named Peter for many years and generously rewarded his services. Practitioners named Stephen and William occasionally served in his retinue, too. Several members of the family also established hospitals and monasteries.

The Beaumonts were powerful in the midland counties. Far to the southwest different generations of the Nonant clan patronized local Devonshire physicians. In the south and east members of the large Chesney family regularly appeared with physicians, especially Robert, bishop of Lincoln from 1148 to 1164. In the north the Lacys, Ilbert and his brother Henry, were served by Lambert the physician for more than three decades. In sickness Henry de Lacy once vowed to found an abbey if he recovered. Accordingly, in 1147 he built Kirkstall in western Yorkshire for the Cistercians, and he spent the next thirty years aiding other monasteries. Geoffrey de Mandeville, earl of Essex, gathered two doctors about him in 1140x1144, but this may have been in his last illness.

The great bishops also patronized physicians. Bishop Roger of Salisbury evidently shared Nigel of Calne's service with the king. Bishop William Warelwast of Exeter was attended by Ralph and by Clarembald, another royal physician. Nigel, the bishop of Ely, Bishop Roger's nephew, associated with two doctors. At different times the bishops of Canterbury, Lincoln, Rochester, Winchester, and York also knew medical attendants, but on the whole, lay lords seem to have been greater patrons. This is rather surprising because bishops generally had the better organized households.

The rewards for medical service could be substantial, but over the years there occurred a decided change in the way these emoluments were granted. The Conqueror was exceptionally generous, even extravagant, in favors to certain physicians, and William Rufus seems to have followed a similar policy. Initially, King Henry was also quite liberal, but his thriftier nature soon asserted itself. The picture is complicated by the fact that some of the earliest practitioners received preferment in Normandy, although they occasionally worked in England. Generally speaking, the shifting rewards paralleled the increasing laicization of the medical profession.

Late eleventh-century physicians were often clerics and two of them became bishops. Gilbert Maminot for Lisieux and John of Tours for Bath. Despite a vow of poverty, monastic physicians could also reap great personal and community rewards from a successful practice. A doctor might become an abbot. More assuredly, the offerings of his grateful patients would enlarge and beautify conventual facilities. Thus, Baldwin was made abbot of Bury in 1065, a year before the Conquest. Faritius, a monk of Malmesbury, became abbot of Abingdon and received innumerable gifts for his house. Ranulf, a royal clerk, entered the Cluniac priory of Montacute and may have eventually become prior there. Hugh, a monk of Winchester, was elected abbot of Chertsey in 1107, although he was not noticeably rewarded thereafter. For the next forty years no English physician who was an ecclesiastic became a bishop or an abbot, until Ailred was elected abbot of Revesby in 1143.

In the beginning lay physicians accumulated large estates, which they carefully bequeathed to their heirs. Argentien, who seems to have been with King William at Hastings Field, was handsomely rewarded with spoils from the defeated foe. He was a cupbearer to the Conqueror and his descendants of many generations displayed three silver cups on their family shield.[44] Even more successful in attaining quick wealth was Nigel medicus, listed in Domesday Book as holding extensive lands in seven counties.[45] Lay physicians continued to prosper under the Conqueror's sons, but there was a marked trend toward rewarding the doctors with money rather than land. Grimbald, for example, served King Henry all his life, but apparently accumulated only thirty-seven hides in six different counties and some city property in Winchester. Gilbert of Falaise, however, acquired considerable capital somewhere, because he was able to offer the exchequer forty-five silver marks for the Nottingham lands and the daughter of John of Monte Caluino. Smaller, but nonetheless impressive, estates were built up by Gervase, Melbethe, Peter, Ralph of Lincoln, and Serlo. Additionally, there were the regular fees for medical treatments, sums that by all accounts were high, even exhorbitant. Indeed, complaints about the supposedly unjustified cost of medical service were loud and persistent throughout this period.

Contrary to the situation elsewhere, Jews did not figure prominently in Anglo-Norman medicine. Only after mid-century can a Jewish practitioner be identified by name. Nevertheless, early London probably did have a Jewish healer. In 1130 its prosperous Hebraic community was fined an enormous penalty—two hundred pounds—for killing a sick man.[46] The circumstances were not specified, but presumably a Christian had sought medical treatment. The magnitude of the assessment suggests that the government sought more than health care regulation in its punishment. Such an amount, for example, could have conveniently cancelled any indebtedness King Henry may have had to the Jews.

Many of the London Jews came from Rouen, where the flourishing, learned Jewish community prided itself on an extraordinarily impressive school.[47] One of these immigrants, Rabbi Joseph (Rubi Gotsce), was a leader of those paying the fine of 1130, and he may well have possessed medical skill. Certainly, the term *rabbi* sometimes implied physician.[48] Moreover, a later Joseph (or Josce), a Jewish physician active in London by at least 1185, was himself the son of a physician.[49] Since the identification of Rabbi Joseph is still rather tentative, he has not been included in the long list of practitioners, although I have a strong feeling he rightly belongs there.

Every so often the curtain of obscurity parts and a bit more is revealed about another physician — and thereby a bit more about all healers. By emphasizing religion, property, and politics, most records inevitably highlight the work of church and government officials or the movements of the rich and the well born and of their attendants. Such evidence usually neglects average folk — women, farmers, merchants, and artisans. Many physicians are likewise ignored, forgotten, or by-passed. Naturally, most healers encountered exclusively local concerns and accordingly achieved only relatively modest reputations, never touching the great events or personalities of the realm. Many quietly worked in monasteries all their lives. Others worthily served the needs of rural areas, caring for peasant families destined, like their healers, to obscurity.

Before examining the careers of eight men who became involved in national affairs, let us look at one rural practitioner who managed to escape complete anonymity — Wulfric of Haselbury. His life had its own fascinations but can also represent something of the routine of his vanished colleagues. In particular, Wulfric's career suggests the multiple roles physicians played in their local communities.

Wulfric was a Saxon hermit and wonder-working prophet. Fortunately, the memory of his holiness and healing remained vivid for three decades after his death and was at last recorded by a monk from a nearby monastery.[50] Wulfric was thus not a typical practitioner, but his unique characteristics were facets of his own personality, not the special advantages of inherited social position or acquired curial status.

Wulfric was born about 1090 into a Somerset family of moderate means, a family nonetheless quite attuned to the pressing need for marketable skills in a changed world where their race was now a subject people. Somehow Wulfric enjoyed the benefits of a good education and learned to speak and write English, French, and Latin fluently. He was ordained a secular priest and served in the diocese of Salisbury, but, by his own admission, devoted as much time to hunting and hawking as to religion.

In his early thirties, after a chance discussion with a beggar, Wulfric experienced a spiritual conversion. In 1125 he decided to become an anchorite and selected for his enclosure the small cell attached to the north side of the parish church at Haselbury Plucknett, a hamlet on the lands of his feudal patron, William Fitz Walter, not far from Montacute Priory. Many other Saxons felt called to similar solitary vocations. The surprise is not only the countless number of men and women who voluntarily chose this demanding life but also the manner in which their literal flight from the world to the wilderness committed them, not to isolation, but to selfless service of others. They were far from being ignorant reclusive rustics, but were, in fact, important community leaders, and many villages would not have survived without them.

Although devoted to prayer, addicted to such ostentatious penance as frequent immersions in cold water, and restricted to the confines of his hermitage, Wulfric was not cut off from the world. He wrote or copied books, made vestments, collected relics, employed a personal scribe, and kept a body servant. Early visitors to his cell included scholars such as Robert Pullen, an Exeter canon and Oxford lecturer, who interpreted one of Wulfric's dreams, and practical innovators such as Rahere, the former courtier who established the great hospital of Saint Bartholomew in Smithfield just outside London.

Wulfric was no plaster saint; he had all the human emotions. On occasion he could be jealous, irascible, and greedy. Despite painful attempts at self-discipline, he could easily lose his temper and roundly curse animals and people who disturbed him; yet most times he was cooperative and generous. He befriended the area clergy, especially the parish priest, a worthy man named Brichtric, who felt awkward because he knew no French. Wulfric contributed to local poor relief and acted as banker for area residents who entrusted their valuables to him for safekeeping. His own skill in languages 'enabled him to arbitrate disputes between Saxon tenants and Norman lords, and he became a bridge between cultures and classes.[51]

To his counseling the anchorite added gifts of prophecy and foreknowledge, and many great figures of the kingdom enlisted his aid in attempts to learn the future. Most visitors came seeking relief from bodily ills, however, and Wulfric gained a national reputation as a healer. Nothing is known of his medical training. Indeed, his designation as a physician (*prophtea pariter medicus erat*) was couched within a flattering description of his appreciation for the psychological dimension of illness.[52] Wulfric evidently considered himself something of an authority on insomnia, and he had particular success with patients suffering problems of sight and speech. His favorite prescription urged patience and prayer—fairly safe advice in many cases—but at other times his techniques were more sensational, sometimes resulting in cures or remissions people called miraculous. (When his own leg became ulcerated and festering, however, he poured hot candle wax on the wound.)

Like many other practitioners Wulfric prospered from his ministrations, and his career offers an unexpected confirmation of William of Malmesbury's strictures against greedy physicians. Grateful patients pressed gifts on the recluse, and he speedily accumulated substantial wealth—gold, silver, precious cloth, vessels, ornaments, and even farm animals. Matters grew so out of hand that at one point he was robbed by his own servant. Another time a belligerent royal official, Drogo de Monci, accused Wulfric of being a trickster and of hoarding vast treasure that rightfully should be impounded by the king. The baron was struck dumb for his impertinence and supposedly only cured sometime later when King Henry, urged on by Queen Adeliza, personally interceded with Wulfric. Thirty years after the anchorite's death, his biographer still felt impelled to justify the unseemly possessions by explaining that they were used to help the poor and obtain church books and vestments.

The Haselbury hermit's connection with the royal court was tangential, but not inconsequential. Henry refused to support his functionary's persecution of the priest and about 1130 even visited Wulfric's Somerset retreat. Their conversation was not recorded, but three years later, when Wulfric learned the king was planning another trip to Normandy, he tactlessly prophesied that Henry would not live to return. When informed of the prediction, the monarch was understandably annoyed and sent a rider to investigate, but the hermit kept to his oracle. Equally bold was Wulfric's public salutation of Stephen of Blois as future king. Moreover, on the very day Henry died in Normandy, Wulfric is said to have reported the king's passing to William Fitz Walter and to have warned him to prepare for coming events. The old king, he observed, would enter paradise because he had sought peace and justice and had built a splendid new abbey at Reading.

Wulfric lived through the troubles of Stephen's reign, but his interests turned from national affairs to his immediate surroundings. He was somewhat critical of the new religious orders, the Austin canons and the Cistercian monks, and he worried about the growing concentration of monasteries in certain locales. He therefore talked his patron out of establishing an Austin priory at Haselbury. Before his death in February 1154, his good works were already noted by the historian Henry of Huntingdon.[53] This writer and others considered Wulfric a saint, but his cult, locally venerated for years, was never recognized by Rome.

At the northern end of the country another holy Saxon healer, Godric of Finchale, also lived a vigorous life of service for others, but likewise remained uncanonized.[54] Godric was born in Norfolk about 1069 and eventually became a prosperous merchant shipowner plying his wares in Scotland, Flanders, and Scandinavia. In middle age he became a tireless pilgrim, visiting Rome three times, the Holy Land twice, and Compostella and Saint-Gilles in Provence, a major shrine for lepers and cripples, at least once. On his second trip to Jerusalem he helped tend the sick at the hospital of Saint John, one of the largest hospitals in the world. It was said to have a capacity of two thousand beds and a death rate of about fifty patients a day.[55] Presumably this was Godric's first introduction to serious medical training. After returning from his last pilgrimage he worked for a while as a gatekeeper at the hospital of Saint Giles in Durham. Finally, in 1110, he became a hermit in Finchale, a lovely spot about three miles from Durham. His sister was a nurse in Durham and eventually another solitary at Finchale.

Like Wulfric, Godric was an accomplished linguist who mediated local quarrels. He kept books and wrote hymns in English, even setting them to music. His life was austere, but it included frequent cold baths, evidently for penitential as well as hygienic reasons. He, too, possessed gifts of prophecy and healing and was consulted about a variety of illnesses. After his long life had ended in 1170, women and children from the neighborhood maintained his cult and prayed for his help.

Godric was more like a paramedic than a trained physician. Yet he further demonstrates the important part hermits and anchorites played in providing health care. In life, their concern, availability, and experience enabled them to help others meet severe crises and unforeseen emergencies. They frequently sensed the psychosomatic ramifications of patients' problems better than regular professionals did. In death, they continued to fill the psychological needs of local people. They were indeed pioneers of later church-sponsored institutions and ultimately of certain types of philanthropy now usually undertaken by public authorities.[56]

A third Saxon and a good friend of Godric, Abbot Ailred of Rievaulx, fared better in the church's tests of sanctity. The charm of his personality may have made part of the difference. However, he also represented the new reform spirit of corporate Cistercian monasticism rather than the older individualistic service of the village hermit. Although painfully ill and therefore a classic case of the physician unable to heal himself, Ailred did help heal others, and in the long view he belongs to the same ascetic, wonder-working tradition as Wulfric. One of the more famous men of his time, Ailred vividly crosses the centuries in his own voluminous writings and in Master Walter Daniel's contemporary biography.

The collective portrayal of all physicians—saints and sinners—paves the way for an examination of those eight special practitioners directly associated with King Henry. They shared many of the finer qualities of their less political colleagues, but encountered additional complexities in their ministrations.

III. HENRICAN
COURT PHYSICIANS

Amidst the cavalcade of soldiers, clerks, prelates, and suppliants who habitually followed the wandering court of King Henry, there were invariably several distinguished physicians. At the end of his life the headstrong lord spurned their sound advice, but until that time he enjoyed the company of medical men, sought them far and wide, and rewarded their special services.

As always, Henry valued his associates for more than one reason. His concern for medicine exhibits the self-interest, manipulation, curiosity, public awareness, and presumptive right that characterize all his activities. Eight practitioners definitely worked for him or his family. In general chronological order these were John of Bath, Ranulf, Clarembald, and Nigel of Calne, all of whom were secular clergymen; Faritius, a monk; Grimbald and Pedro Alfonso, two foreign laymen; and Serlo of Arundel, also a clerk. A physician named Mark had vague links with the royal court but cannot yet be directly related to the king.

Several among the eight doctors proudly announced their professional association with the royal family. Others attended the king but evidently found a pretentious title unnecessary. Still others worked at court, more in a religious or bureaucratic than a medical capacity. Collectively they illustrate the range of talent which could be consulted but individually each practitioner achieved his success in quite a different way.

John was a holdover from the awkward days of King William Rufus, and, like that puzzling ruler, he, too, gained an unfavorable reputation. Age would eventually mellow some of his rougher qualities, but John was often excessively hard on his subordinates. He was sometimes called John of Villula, sometimes John of Tours, but most often John of Bath, after the diocese he governed for thirty-four years.

Born in Tours, John was said to have had little formal training but much practical experience in medicine. While this typically caustic judgment from the monastic historian William of Malmesbury demonstrates that physicians were expected to possess classroom learning, it could have a further critical intent. As well as ridiculing John's alleged on-the-job training, such a description might also characterize the old-style pragmatic instruction once offered at Salerno, and probably at Montpellier and Marmoutier, in the years before theoretical studies triumphed under the banner of Islamic scholarship. Although he subsequently toned down his written opinion, Malmesbury clearly did not like John. The monk's original manuscript had characterized the physician-prelate as silly, unstable, and prone to drink and had claimed that he made a great deal of money from his practice. A revised version, dating from perhaps fifteen years later, merely stated that John began his reforms too hastily. That much, at least, was true.[1]

John was probably one of the physicians at the deathbed of the Conqueror.[2] Thereafter he served William Rufus as chaplain for about a year, and in 1088 he was raised to the bishopric of Wells. It was a handsome reward, granted perhaps because the king considered him a kindred spirit. In the new diocese John's immediate concern was to find lucrative positions for his brother, Hildebert, and his nephew. In achieving this, he disrupted the Saxon cathedral canons, violated their chapter statutes, pulled down their conventual buildings, and forced them to locate other lodgings. The fuss was almost pointless, for within two years his attention turned from Wells to Bath, the ruined but more advantageous town that he had just purchased from the king for five hundred pounds.

John arrogantly transferred his episcopal seat to the abbey at Bath and made it a cathedral priory. Then he expansively laid out an enormous new basilica, created a school, endowed a library, and refitted two of the derelict Roman baths to develop their medical potential. The investment was a great success.[3] Soon, sick people from all over England flocked to Bath, trying to wash away their infirmities. Poets and chroniclers praised its hot springs, and a prominent local baron quickly built a leper hospital outside town.[4] The new reign offered additional opportunities for the calculating bishop. John immediately sought confirmation of his property from King Henry as well as from Duke Robert of Normandy — just in case there was a change of leadership.

Perhaps because of this half-hearted support, John never gained any special intimacy with Henry. The bishop's abrasive personality may also have put off the new ruler. Like any magnate, at regular intervals Bishop John attested royal writs and executed royal commands but no unusual favors came his way. An insensitive individual, he was an intellectual nonetheless. Even William of Malmesbury grudgingly admitted that John rejoiced "in the society of learned men."[5] One of these associates was undoubtedly Adelard of Bath, and the great naturalist probably owes an unacknowledged debt to this rough-hewn bishop for a start in his career. The prelate lived to a ripe old age. In 1122, right after Christmas dinner, he suffered a heart attack and died within four days.

John of Bath may well have maintained part of his medical practice all his life. Decades after the bishop's death, Henry of Huntingdon still remembered that he had been a physician as well as a bishop.[6]

Ranulf the physician had a far more generous personality than John and he could boast of a professional and personal intimacy with the king which always eluded the bishop. Paradoxically, Ranulf's very success made him yearn for a far different life. He tired of flattery, rivalry, and patronage, like several other courtiers of Henry's circle. Rather early in the reign, convinced of higher ideals, he threw over wealth and honors and entered an obscure monastery on the Welsh frontier. For his new vocation Ranulf chose to enter Malpas Priory in Monmouthshire, a cell of Montacute Priory in Somerset, one of the Cluniac foundations much favored by the court.

As a royal physician Ranulf had amassed a small estate in Monmouth, perhaps his native area. His possessions consisted of some thirty-three acres of land, chapels, mills, buildings, fisheries, and rights to sea wreckage; all these he gave to Malpas with the consent of his lord, Robert de Haia, and of the king himself. Proclaiming himself physician of the king (*Ranulfus, domini H[enrici] Regis medicus*), Ranulf enshrined his gift in a long charter and signed it with his own seal. (His use of a personal device is interesting, since later physicians would also refer to their own seals.) Although the text of Ranulf's donation was badly jumbled when copied into the Montacute Priory cartulary, the significance of his title was not lost on contemporaries. In 1132 the phrase "physician of King Henry" was repeated by Earl Robert of Gloucester in each of his two confirmations of Ranulf's original grant.[7]

Although he sought cloistered obscurity, Ranulf may have attracted considerable attention. By 1112 a prior of Montacute named Ranulf appears in the records and he may well have been the physician transferred from Malpas. Certainly the royal court continued to favor Montacute for some years. One of the principal benefactors was a royal chancellor, confusingly also named Ranulf but clearly distinct from the physician and the prior. Lands belonging to Grimbald, the court physician, further enhanced Montacute's endowment. Evidently the king had once had great plans for the monastery, but later turned his attention to founding Reading Abbey.[8]

Clarembald was another man in the west country with spiritual and medical training who proudly, almost boastfully served King Henry. This practitioner never settled on a single method of satisfactorily identifying himself, however, and is known to have described his occupational status as physician, physician and chaplain, chaplain of the king, and clerk. Clarembald was a self-conscious literary stylist, an author, a bibliophile, and a collector of miracle stories. He died about 1133, so his career covered most of Henry's reign; but rather than follow his lord about the realm, he seems to have concentrated his activities in London and Devon.[9]

These two places do not exactly represent a separation of local and national, or eccleciastical and civil, responsibilities. In fact, rather than attend court in the east, the physician worked with the bishops of London, the canons of Saint Paul's, and the monks of Westminster. Moreover, in the west, Exeter was near the center rather than the periphery of royal affairs. Like most towns, it had its castle, schools, churches, monasteries, mints, markets, and water mills. Its Norman cathedral, erected in the early twelfth century, symbolized life and driving progress. The town's real distinction, however, derived from its academic community. Men like Robert Pullen, Master Odo (who may have been one of Abelard's pupils in Paris), Honorius of Autun, and Master Algar, dean of Bodmin and Bishop of Coutances (1132–1151), were Clarembald's colleagues, and for a while they created an unusually vigorous intellectual atmosphere. Several of these men had connections with the famous French cathedral school of Laon, and it was to that city that Bishop William Warelwast sent his nephew, presumably after preliminary training in Exeter.[10]

Bishop William was the towering personage in town. A Norman by birth, he was one of the most influential diplomats of his era, and a prototype of the professional civil servant. If his cathedral chapter was noted for its intellectuals, his governmental entourage bristled with ambitious clerks, like Bernard the king's scribe, a Saxon from Cornwall who used his court position to reestablish the lost fortunes of his family. The bishop is a particularly intriguing figure, as he was not only Clarembalds's diocesan but probably his patient as well. For more than fifty years, despite increasing adversity, Warelwast faithfully served as confidant to William Rufus and Henry. Between 1095 and 1105 he made at least five trips to Rome as royal envoy and then three more between 1116 and 1120.

A crusty, indefatigable ambassador, William was not without shortcomings. Evidently he once brutally criticized an earlier bishop of Exeter for remaining in office after going blind. The chroniclers therefore found it ironic that Warelwast lost his own sight almost eighteen years before his death. Needless to say, he did not himself resign but continued his travels despite his infirmity becoming the butt of cruel jokes in the Roman curia. Although his health was otherwise good, Bishop William once journeyed to Rome accompanied by Hugh, the abbot-physician of Chertsey, and he regularly kept his own doctors, such as Clarembald and a certain Ralph.[11]

Clarembald's name appears on five charters, but none of these deeds directly involved the king. His announcement in 1128 that he was the king's chaplain was, however, supported by an exchequer pardon in 1130 for twenty-two shillings for lands in Devon. This indicates that he had a modest but comfortable country estate as a reward for, or in right of, some definite royal service.[12]

Clarmebald was probably the attending physician for another imperious prelate, Richard of Beaumais, the bishop of London (1108–27). This ambitious churchman exercised wide governmental authority in the west country until he suffered a paralyzing stroke in 1124. Recognizing the beckoning of eternity he spent the remaining years of his life trying to remedy the bad effects of certain earlier decisions. Shortly before his death he drafted a series of writs returning various properties to the churches from which he had taken them. One witness to these deathbed provisions was Clarembald the clerk, probably Clarembald of Exeter.[13]

Besides the local teachers, royal scribes, and curial bishops with whom he frequently associated, Clarembald was also friendly with one of the greatest poets of the age, Hildebert of Lavardin. This prolific writer was familiar with English conditions. He had visited the country twice around the turn of the century and later sent several of his brightest clerks to work there. Between 1118 and 1125 Clarembald wrote up a series of miracles which had occurred at Exeter Cathedral and sent the description to Bishop Hildebart at Le Mans. He received no reply. Undaunted, Clarembald prepared a revised edition and posted it, too. Somewhat embarrassed, Hildebart then answered with a florid, but rather vague, note apologizing for his tardiness. Presumably a messenger returned one of the tracts annotated with Hildebert's specific suggestions. Unfortunately, neither treatise has survived. One wonders if Clarembald employed much clinical judgment in describing symptoms, illnesses, and cures. A short poem merely listing some miracles at Exeter is extant and may be another of Clarembald's works, or a synopsis of his earlier effort.[14]

Another fragment of the physician's correspondence may also be intact. A talented, testy, controversial monk of Westminister Abbey, Osbert of Clare, once corresponded with an unidentified Clarembald. His letter implies that the recipient had some supervision over a religious community. (It would be interesting to know if this was a hospital.) The case for identifying the addressee with Clarembald medicus is fairly strong. He had once attested for Westminister. Moreover, in his letter Osbert made exactly the same flattering pun about his friend's name — Clarembald equals Clarusvalde equals very illustrious — that Hildebert had once made about Clarembald of Exeter.

Osbert's petulant, self-centered epistle complained that everyone was neglecting him and that he felt like a shorn Samson in sickness and distress. Toward the end he says that if "Dom Nicholas has gathered any sacred flowers for me, pray send them by this messenger." The reference could be to the brother of Bernard, the royal scribe, Nicholas, a canon of Merton and a scribe himself, who was active in Cornwall affairs. Medicine was not discussed in this note, but as a pyschological profile of its author, the letter might have intrigued a physician recipient.[15]

As one of twenty-four canons of Exeter, Clarembald would have received a prebend and a yearly stipend of four pounds, but he also had considerable private wealth, probably derived from his medical practice and governmental service. He lived apart from the canons in a large townhouse that fronted on South Street and evidently extended the entire length of the southern side of that road. The property included an oratory dedicated to Saint Radegund. This obscure French queen was a patron of lepers and hospitals and was especially venerated in Tours. She was also the subject of one of Hildebert's studies. The odd devotional practice, employed in Clarembald's day, of sick persons offering to a shrine a wax candle as long as their combined height and waist measurements dates back to Radegund's time.[16]

One book from the physician's library may have survived. The name Clarembald was inscribed in an early twelfth-century copy of Bede's exegetical commentary, *De Tabernaculo*. This long, unillustrated biblical treatise discussed Moses' plans for the new temple, including descriptions of the altar, the ark of the covenant', and the functions of priests. Although a costly and unusual possession for a private individual, copies of the treatise could be found in many monastic and cathedral libraries.[17]

Clarembald died, apprarently without heirs, shortly before July, 1133. At the consecration of the new minister, Bishop Warelwast directed that "the house wherein Clarembald had dwelt until the day of his death" should be granted to Plympton Priory.[18] The prelate had established this daughter house of Merton Priory for Austin canons about a dozen years earlier. Other parts of Clarembald's property passed, for unknown reasons, to a Walter Fitz Drogo.

Like Clarembald, Nigel of Calne divided his service between the king and a powerful bishop. His traces in the contemporary records, however, are extremely ambiguous, because several physicians bore the name Nigel and many bureaucrats identified themselves with the small village of Calne. The Conqueror had rewarded one Nigel medicus so extravagantly that in 1086 he held estates in nine different counties, including the church and royal manor of Calne, in Wiltshire. This wealthy practitioner was hardly a friend of the church, but his exact contemporary, Nigel, the physician of Earl Robert of Shrewsbury, was a clerk. This particular Nigel held a benefice in Shropshire and died in 1094x1098. A third, and most complex, Nigel medicus was the earliest occupant of the prebend of Mora in the chapter of Saint Paul's Cathedral.

Nigel of Mora did not cut a great figure in the cathedral muniments. His sole appearance in a thirteenth-century catalog listed him as the first holder of the prebend.[19] Unfortunately, there is no satisfactory way to date when he gained or lost this rewarding post. His successor was Bishop Everard — that is Everard of Calne — who was the bishop of Norwich from 1121 to 1145. The episcopal designation suggests that Everard may have received the benefice after his consecration, because other canons who became bishops were usually not listed with their titles in this catalog. Everard in turn was succeeded by his nephew, William, who first appeared as a canon between 1108 and 1138. Thus, at Saint Paul's, a Nigel medicus received the Mora prebend prior to 1138, probably long before then.

Several authorities believe domesday Nigel was also Nigel of Mora. This seems quite unlikely to me. In 1086 the Domesday tenant-in-chief was already an important individual, but prebendary Nigel seems to have been just rising in the world.[20]

To confuse matters even more, there were two additional Nigels from the same time and area — Nigel of Calne and Nigel, the nephew of Bishop Roger of Salisbury. Could either of them have been a physician? The case for the bishop's nephew is far too weak since a great deal is known about him, and the information does not support such an assumption. He studied at Laon before 1112 with his brother Alexander, the future bishop of Lincoln, became royal treasurer under King Henry, and was selected bishop Ely, serving from 1133 to 1169. If he had pursued medical training, surely some of the writers and officials who knew him would have alluded to it.

On the other hand, Nigel of Calne, a royal chaplain and a canon of Salisbury Cathedral, closely fits the Mora doctor's profile. This Nigel's habit of describing himself as "of Calne," seemingly a family practice, preceded his acceptance of the important benefice created just for him. Indeed, between 1107 and 1116 King Henry not only granted the church of Calne and all its appurtenances to the Sarum chapter in order to endow the new canonry of Calne, he also personally nominated Nigel "of Calne" as its first occupant.[21] The prebend entailed the village church and its privileges and considerable rights in the royal forest, including two horses a year, an unusual extra stripend. Henry's detailed personal interest suggests that he had a special regard for this Nigel or an exceptional desire to reward some service.

On the surface, however, Nigel of Calne's governmental career seems quite ordinary. He traveled extensively with the king's court and acted as a chaplain. Most likely he was also a chancery clerk, who drafted and recorded documents. He never called attention to his medical skill and rarely used any title, except once, when he witnessed a royal writ as Nigel of Calne, chaplain. Oddly, his ministerial attestations were all made in Normandy.[22]

In addition to this civil employment, Nigel of Calne fulfilled his commitments to the Salisbury bishop and chapter. In 1108x1110 he was one of a large number of barons and churchmen, including Roger of Salisbury, who counseled Bishop William Giffard of Winchester in a complex land dispute.[23] In 1122 he witnessed Bishop Roger's confirmation of the creation of another Sarum prebend. Like everyone else, Nigel was anxious to advance the careers of his relatives; thus, in 1130 he paid the exchequer one silver mark for an unspecified debt of his nephew William.[24]

Nigel of Calne's association with the Salisbury diocese and the government bureaucracy was duplicated by Everard of Calne's similar occupational pursuits. Before he became bishop of Norwich, Everard had been an archdeacon of Sarum and had also worked in the royal chancery. Increasingly, government policy supported civil servants by offering them lucrative benefices at major churches, such as Saint Paul's, Saint Martin-le-Grand, and Waltham Holy Cross. Not surprisingly, the men who worked most closely with the viceroy, Roger of Salisbury, sometimes received a living both in his diocese and in other metropolitan centers where they worked. By holding more than one ecclesiastical benefice, Everard and Nigel both became pluralists, a regrettable distinction they shared with their episcopal master.[25]

Since both Everard and Nigel of Calne had a nephew named William, they were probably brothers as well as successive prebendaries at Saint Paul's. In fact, Everard was consolidating his late father's affairs in 1130 and William's debt may have involved the same inheritance.[26] Other people calling themselves "of Calne" can be found in the pipe roll of 1130 and among the retainers of the bishops of Norwich.[27] All of this evidence strengthens the case for equating the physician Nigel of Mora with the bureaucrat Nigel of Calne. Whether or not the Domesday Nigel, the Shropshire Nigel, and the London-Salisbury Nigel were members of the same Calne family must remain conjectural.

The identification of Nigel of Mora with Nigel of Calne closes one puzzling gap in the long chain of Anglo-Norman practitioners. Hitherto no physician could closely be associated with Roger of Salisbury. Naturally, the bishop knew the doctors who surrounded the king, but no medical man had had any special attachment to his own episcopal or viceregal household. Yet it is almost inconceivable that this unique royal minister, who so closely shared Henry's administrative responsibility and his outlook on life, would not also have mirrored his lord's fascination with medicine. Roger's prominent support of hospitals can easily be demonstrated, and now his working relationship with at least one physician is also evident. It is disappointing that Nigel's medical experience was highlighted only in London and not in his travels with the king or the bishop, but the familiar pattern of healers only sporadically revealing their profession is thus repeated.

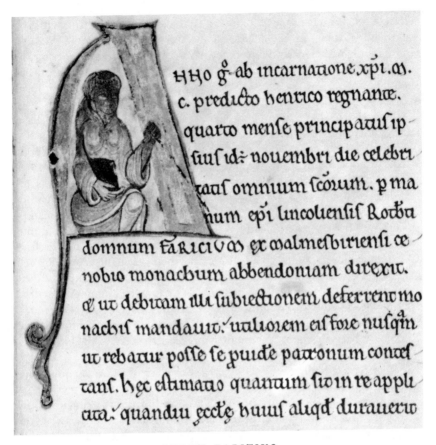

ABBOT FARITIUS

The most influential of King Henry's physicians was Faritius of Abingdon. When that monastery's records were recopied before 1170, an artist added this likeness of the famed Italian practitioner within the letter A. The text reports that on November 1, 1100 Faritius, a monk of Malmesbury, was chosen abbot of Abindgon. By permission of the British Library, Ms. Cotton Claudius C IX, fo. 144.

The foregoing men worked for the king in the capacity of chaplain, and official as much as medical practitioner but Faritius of Abingdon regularly treated the royal household. According to all accounts he was a most engaging individual—good conversationist, avid bibliophile, talented author, master builder, and successful fund raiser. These varied interests not only suggest why people were so attracted to him but also reflect the interdisciplinary, unspecialized nature of learning in the early twelfth century. Indeed, one suspects that Faritius sometimes excelled more through his charming bedside manner than through any exceptional curative skill.

Born in Arezzo, in Tuscany, this physician first appears in Britain as the cellarer—part quartermaster, part guestmaster, part infirmarian—of Malmesbury Abbey in 1078. Next, at the very dawn of Henry's reign, a young monk at the ancient and somewhat decrepit abbey of Abingdon, in Berkshire, had a vision directing him to urge his brothers to elect Faritius as their new abbot. The doctor must have had a splendid reputation, for royal approval came quickly, and he was consecrated on November 1, 1100.[28]

Some scholars have speculated that as an Italian, Faritius would have studied medicine at Salerno. If he did—and no evidence supports such a contention—his master would most likely have been that city's archbishop, Alfans, a notable physician, humanist, and scholar whose medical writings embodied the traditional, pre-Arabic, classical learning. Salerno was renowned, even criticized, for its concentration on clinical technique rather than theoretical instruction, but the epitomizing works of Alfans mark a shift toward more theoretical studies. His most famous pupil was the former Moslem merchant, Constantine the African, who learned Latin as well as Christianity from Alafans about 1077, and then spent the remaining ten years of his life at nearby Monte Cassino translating important medical texts from Arabic. That famous Benedictine abbey had been a center of medical learning even before Constantine's arrival, and it is in some ways more logical to think of Faritius the monk as a product of Monte Cassino than of Salerno. Whatever school he attended, his teachers were of the older, pre-Arabic tradition.

Before he left Malmesbury Abbey, Faritius composed a biography of its great patron, Saint Aldhelm (d. 709). Although peppered with interjections concerning the hero's sanctity, the tract is a valid piece of research. A brief prologue justifies antiquarian investigation and reminds readers that the Evangelist Luke was also a physician.[29] Decades later, after Faritius's death, William of Malmesbury composed his own life of Aldhelm. He was rather condescending toward the earlier study, claiming that, as a foreigner, Faritius did not really understand the Saxon language and the early sources and that he had consequently drawn some improper conclusions. Saintly Bishop Osmund of Salisbury (1076–99), who was also born abroad wrote his own story of Aldhelm, but William did not mention it. Malmesbury's criticism seems unwarranted and his motivation suspicious, particularly since differences between his and Faritius's works now appear so small.[30]

After all, Faritius was certainly the most famous monk to have been at Malmesbury in many years. Moreover, William studied medicine, and it is conceivable that Faritius had been his earliest instructor, although the other house physician, Gregory, is a more likely candidate. In any event, throughout all his books William's references to Faritius were curiously infrequent, brief, and ambivalent. For example, William did record the abbot's death in 1117, yet he included, not his own praise, but a poem in Faritius's honor by another Malmesbury monk, Peter, who was mainly impressed by the physician's famous patients and luxurious church decorations.[31] Fortunately, anonymous chroniclers at Abingdon more eagerly preserved significant details about Faritius's later life.

At the new monastery Faritius seems to have broadened his medical practice, especially in the beginning. In 1101, when Queen Matilda was expecting her first child, a royal command went out to the doctors, presumably a good number, to be near at hand to care for her and to make known her prognosis. Of these healers, Faritius was the most important, and he was ably seconded by his fellow countryman and cherished friend, Grimbald.[32] The lying-in took place at Winchester. Duke Robert of Normandy, who was then invading England, chivalrously marched away from the town when he learned the queen was there. (It was the least he could do as her godfather.) The birth was probably very difficult; in any event, the child did not survive infancy. Matilda was exceedingly grateful for Faritius's assistance and became one of his staunchest supporters. During her lifetime the rewards never stopped flowing over Abingdon. Faritius probably also assisted at the births of her other two children, William and Matilda. The king, who declared great personal confidence in Faritius, usually followed only his prescriptions.[33]

Faritius was a great favorite not only of the royal family but also, as one writer strangely put it, of all the older people of England.[34] The commentator was at a loss to explain the strong effect the abbot's words, personality, and techniques had upon individuals. Patients from such families as the de Veres, Fitz Hamons, and Crispins found relief at the Berkshire abbey and left behind expensive reminders of their gratitude. Even when the treatments were unsuccessful, the relatives were grateful. Aubrey de Vere's sick son, Geoffrey, at first seemed to improve under Faritius's care. Unfortunately, he died shortly thereafter, of a different malady, and was buried in the abbey. On his death bed Geoffrey granted the monks the tithes of a church, a gift his father subsequently enlarged. Aubrey made the grant to thank the monks for his son's care and to prepare for his own salvation, because, as the chronicler recording the donation wrote, "there is no medicine against death."[35] Eventually the Vere gift formed the nucleus of a new priory at Colne, in Essex, which became the traditional burial ground of the family and its dependents.[36]

Robert Fitz Hamon was probably another terminal patient. If he consulted Abbot Faritius about the wound he sustained in 1105, his relief was only temporary, for he lingered in considerable discomfort until 1107. Yet it was apparently during that interval that Faritius, as "Pharisyus," attested two of Robert's grants to the church of Cranbourne.[37] Such attestatioins on the abbot's part were extremely rare, but numerous donors cane to the convent to solemnize gifts, to arrange for burial rights, or to return lands expropriated in earlier days.[38] Some were accompanied by their own physicians, and Faritius, who seems to have made diagnostic analysis a lifelong specialty, evidently had many acquaintances in the medical fraternity.[39]

There was a certain eminence to his practice. While other doctors, like his friend Grimbald, traveled with their lords or the king, Faritius kept close to Abingdon. Although he would rush to judicial sessions to defend his abbey's privileges, many royal and ecclesiastical ceremonies passed without his attendance.[40] Even though Faritius rarely attested royal, or baronial, decrees, the king's largesse remained unabated, and Abingdon and its abbot appear to have received more gifts than any other religious house. After Faritius's death the transformation was shocking. The benefactions immediately stopped, and abbots were actually hauled into court to defend past privileges and to pay heavy fines.

While Faritius lived, however, the monastery enjoyed unrivaled prosperity. The number of monks increased from twenty-eight to eighty. New cloisters, towers, and chapels were built, and supplies and carpenters for the work were brought in from Wales. Tapestries were hung and rooms were lavishly decorated. Resident scribes busily copied all types of volumes, including "many books of medicine [*de physica*]."[41] The abbot corresponded in friendly fashion with learned scholars, such as Theobald of Etampes, the "master of Oxford," who wrote about the necessity of infant baptism, a subject of debate between the two men.[42] Precious relics arrived from as far away as Constantinople, and a grammar school was organized for lay students, including royal bastards.[43]

The abbot was an important baron, a major tenant-in-chief, because Abingdon had been assigned a high military service quota of thirty knights at the Conquest. In order to support these men, lands were granted out as military fiefs. But over the years, the vassals thus enfeoffed tended to neglect their obligations to the abbot and assumed a type of tenurial independence. As a result, Faritius devoted much time to regaining control of such alienated lands. A shrewd businessman, he usually attained "his own will either by prayer or by price."[44] The victories were actually somewhat illusory, however, for he was more successful in receiving new gifts than in controlling old tenants. Numerous stern but repetitive royal writs testify to his difficulties in reasserting abbatial dominion.[45]

In the course of such negotiations, however, Faritius became quite skilled in the law. He was among the first to obtain exemption from the 1110 feudal aid collected for the marriage of the king's daughter. He was also one of the earliest appellants to Domesday Book, which was then kept in the Winchester treasury, and one of the original beneficiaries of the new writ of right.[46] Always attuned to the realities of a situation and never backward in using his friends, Faritius sometimes arranged to have his problems adjudicated by the queen's court while the king was in Normandy.[47]

The abbot's career was not an unqualified triumph, however. His monas-

tery grew in members, buildings, and wealth, but Faritius's medical responsibilities, fund raising, and constant litigation gradually isolated him from
his monks. He even had a separate dining room erected for himself, and
there were complaints of the disparity of food in the two halls.[48]

In 1114 Henry decided to confer the highest honor in his power on Abbot
Faritius by making him archbishop of Canterbury. Saintly old Anselm had
died in 1109, and the king had happily pocketed Canterbury's revenues during the intervening years. He was clearly in no great rush to elevate his physician, but he surely considered Faritius a suitable choice. Others, however,
did not. The Canterbury election of 1114 thereby became a surprisingly
complicated event.[49]

Despite his great reputation, some people thought Faritius might be too
strict a reformer. Others complained that an equally qualified Norman
ought to be chosen—an oddly chauvinistic argument considering the Italian
births of Lanfranc and Anselm. An even more devisive argument concerned
the particular ecclesiastical status of the candidate. A long line of monks,
like Faritius, had occupied the primatial chair of all England, but change
was in the wind. Some powerful curial bishops, led by Roger of Salisbury
and Robert Bloet of Lincoln, proposed that it was time for a secular clerk to
become archbishop, and this was probably the nub of the opposition to
Faritius. However, Bishops Roger and Robert also made the extraordinary assertion that they opposed the abbot because it was unseemly for a man who
had examined the urine of women to become episcopal ruler of all England.
Whether this was a coarse joke, a fatuous excuse, or a superficial but perceptive summary of current informed sentiment, the discussion could hardly
have pleased the king or the queen. One wonders what John of Bath said.
Certainly there were plenty of precedents for prelate-physicians.

To all appearances the two bishops had no personal reasons for opposing
Faritius's candidacy. Robert Bloet had enthroned him as abbot, and Roger of
Salisbury, his diocesan bishop, had frequently lent his powerful support to
Abingdon's never-ending quest for additional endowment. Both men, however, may well have been in touch with the forward drift of ecclesiastical
thought that seriously questioned the propriety of monks practicing as paid
physicians. For example, the great French contemporary, bishop Hildebert
of Lavardin, had poetically observed that physicians were continually exposed to three great temptations: women, ambition, and greed.[50]

The church's objection was not so much to the requirements and practice
of medicine as to the wealth accumulated at the expense of others by clergymen, especially monks vowed to poverty and pledged to withdrawal from
the secular world. Faritius may therefore have been both an outstanding example of financial success in medicine and an early sacrificial casualty in the
church's ongoing hierarchical reform.[51]

King Henry did not need a horoscope or a urinalysis color chart to tell how the prognosis for this election was developing. He could have forced his will upon the clergy, but the Investiture Controversy had made him wary of unnecessary quarrels with the church. Furthermore, his own personality never inclined him to initiate struggles for uncertain results, particularly when he was opposed by two of his own principal advisers. Therefore he quietly backed down and substituted a compromise candidate, Ralph of Rochester.

Abbot Faritius gracefully retreated to Abingdon, but his fortunes continued to decline. The very opulence of the abbey now rose up to haunt him. Many monks had never appreciated that his secular and feudal obligations necessitated a separate and rather ostentatious household. The nasty difficulties about refectory expenses also worsened to such a degree that the king eventually decided to send a commission to investigate. The panel rather awkwardly consisted of Archbishop Ralph, Bishop Roger of Salisbury, and Hugh of Buckland, sheriff of Berkshire and one of Faritius's own vassals. The accused abbot vigorously defended his policies and achievements before this trio and before his own monks. Although his actions were generally upheld, it must have been a humiliating experience.[52]

Faritius died soon afterward of indigestion, an ironic turn of fate in light of the quarrels within his community about dining facilities. His life's end exhibited the same organizational grasp that had characterized his whole career. Recognizing his symptoms, and perhaps no longer relishing life, Faritius prophesied his own death and asked that notice be sent to Bishop Roger and to Abbot Edulf of Malmesbury, his old abbey. He left valuable gifts on the high altar of his church—ormaments, vestments, endowments for books, alms for the poor, and funds to heat the sick rooms—and threatened excommunication of anyone who disturbed his bequests. How a monk who had taken a vow of poverty had accumulated such treasure was apparently never asked. Faritius's last words, on February 23, 1117, were said to echo the Psalmist: "Lord, I have loved the beauty of thy house." There was much truth, and even double meaning, in his final sentiment.[53]

The influence of Faritius lived on in the person of his close friend and professional associate Grimbald. Whether or not these two comrades first met in northern Italy or in central England, they evidently knew one another before jointly assisting Queen Matilda. Furthermore, from 1101, as signatory to Matilda's first gift to Abingdon, until 1117, almost half of Grimbald's attestations involved royal grants for the abbot or his convent. Thereafter his contact, like Henry's generosity, ceased abruptly. Grimbald was no mere shadow of Faritius, however. He was a layman who raised a family, and he outlived his friend by twenty years. He traveled throughout England beside his royal patients for more than three decades and, at least in 1113, 1126, and 1130, accompanied the king to Normandy.[54]

Royal favors came slowly but faithfully. Sometime after 1115 Grimbald's family acquired a house in Winchester near the royal palace, and by 1130

Grimbald was tenant-in-chief, holding lands directly from the king in five different counties.[55] He seems to have helped endow Montacute Priory in Somerset, the monastery that frequently fed Wulfric and occasionally housed Ranulf. Grimbald may also have aided Colne Priory, in Essex, the dependent cell of Abingdon originally founded as an expression of gratitude by one of Faritius's patients.[56]

Grimbald died before 1138, leaving a widow, Atselina, and a daughter, Emma, who arranged to transfer the inheritance to her husband, Walter Martel.[57] She may have been an only child, because the fief her father held from Simon, bishop of Worcester reverted back to that prelate rather than staying in the physician's family. (One wonders what service Grimbald performed for this fief.)[58]

It is not known whether Grimbald wrote books, collected relics, or recorded miracles. Although he represented the wave of the future, he probably would have remained totally obscure were it not for one vivid incident that proves him an acute observer of human nature. The chronicler John of Worcester, who was himself quite interested in scientific phenomena, once chanced to visit Winchcombe Abbey while Grimbald was there and heard the physician relate a detailed account of three nightmares the old king had endured in Normandy a few years earlier, in 1130. Grimbald evidently savored this gossip, and John, captivated by the story, later carefully sketched these dreams in his own book. Together with a well-executed drawing of a rough Channel crossing, they are among the earliest examples of secular manuscript illumination. Grimbald's presence at Winchcombe in the early 1130s incidentally raises the possibility that he may not have been part of Henry's retinue during the last, fatal visit to Normandy in 1133-35.[59]

According to the physician's report, Henry first dreamed that he was surrounded by crowds of yelling peasants, who gnashed their teeth and shook scythes and pitchforks in his face. Later he had a vision of mail-clad knights brandishing their swords at him. Finally, bishops and abbots appeared armed with croziers and charters. At each visitation the old ruler jumped from his bed naked, grabbed his sword, shouted at the phantoms, and thrashed about the room, chasing out his frightened guards. Either the nightmares reappeared on succeeding nights or there was some interval between each dream, for in the commotion Grimbald secretly made his way into the the bedchamber and hid himself in a corner to witness his lord's distress. Henry later told him the whole story and asked for an interpretation.

Having gained the king's confidence in this difficult matter, Grimbald wisely attempted some calm, psychological counseling. Unfortunately, his interpretation of the dreams was not recorded. Contemporary medical lore claimed that dreams originated when vapors from the stomach ascended the veins to the brain. Grimbald seemed to be searching for a deeper cause. Indeed, the chronicler likened him to Daniel assisting Nebuchadnezzar and pointed out that the physician similarly advised his lord to undertake a curative series of almsgiving, prayer, and good works.

Grimbald rightly surmised that the king's conscience was troubling him. The content of the dreams was rather ordinary, as such things go, but the extraordinary vividness made a lasting impression on everyone. William of Malmesbury once claimed that Henry was a heavy sleeper whose rest was usually interrupted only by fits of snoring.[60] The Worcester chronicler, perhaps echoing Grimbald's analysis, speculated that it was worry over having imposed high taxes which disturbed the king on this occasion.

Henry's nocturnal frights had a troubled history. In fact, some years earlier his own chamberlain and servants had actually tried to assassinate him while he slept.[61] More recently the king consulted Wulfric of Haselbury, a renowned psychic as well as physician. The visions of threatening farmers, prelates, and soldiers which occurred in Normandy in the summer of 1130 may have sprung from some purely local complaint there, but, more likely, they were related to the general state of the entire Anglo-Norman realm. It was certainly not a good year in England. The weather was dreadful. There was disease among human beings and cattle, and a large part of Rochester burned to the ground. Even more unsettling, Geoffrey de Clinton, an important justice, sheriff, and long-time treasury official, was charged with high treason. In an apparently unrelated incident, several other sheriffs were dismissed from office. Also, a serious dispute erupted at Saint Bartholomew's hospital and priory, and the brothers there rebelled against Rahere, their somewhat secretive founder-prior. In London people were accusing the Jews of murdering a sick man. In Normandy Henry's daughter, his only legitimate heir, was quarreling with her new husband, and her succession to England's crown, should anything happen to Henry, was still questionable.

The troubled king had little peace, and within twelve months he hurried back to England. He was seriously ill at Windsor during Christmas, 1132, and it is probably no accident that several of his gifts to hospitals came in the period immediately following his recovery.

John of Worcester's sketches of the suffering king deserve some attention. Next to each of the three panels of the dreaming sovereign and his threatening visitors sits a long-robed, bearded figure examining small vials and a tiny tablet or booklet. Undoubtedly this is Grimbald the physician observing the king's dreams and later holding a glass bottle of his urine to the light, consulting a color chart, and checking for vapors or excessive humors. These pictures are the oldest portrait of any identifiable practitioner. Since John knew Grimbald, they presumably are fairly accurate likenesses.

The exquisitely graceful manner in which the physician's long, slender fingers caress the bottle is one of the hallmarks of late Romanesque illustration. The gestures are not fanciful, however, for physicians were known to hang at their waists little folded booklets that could be consulted for quick

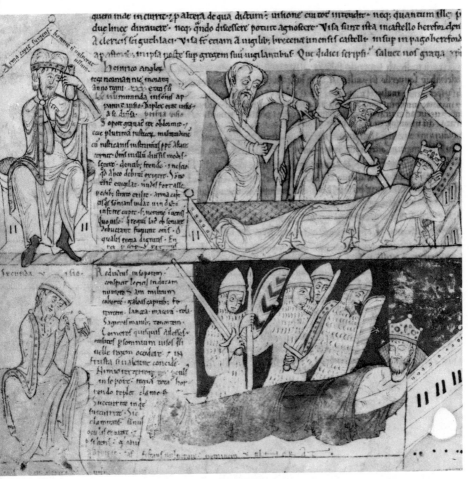

GRIMBALD MEDICUS

as sketched by John of Worcester

In 1130 King Henry dreamed that he was besieged by angry peasants, knights, and churchmen, and he consulted Grimbald about his troubles. The physician told the chronicler John of Worcester, who recorded the incident about 1140. His lightly tinted drawings are among the oldest secular narrative illustrations, and the three views of Grimbald are the only contemporary portraits of an identifiable practitioner. On the facing page of this manuscript Grimbald holds a chart as the king dreams of complaining bishops and abbots. By permission of the President and Fellows of Corpus Christi College, Oxford, Ms. CCC 157, fo. 382.

diagnosis.[62] In some ways the scene is quite modern, not unlike a psychiatrist's office: the patient on the couch, the doctor seated along side, and the dream somewhere in the air between them.

It is quite a leap from Grimbald's unusual experiences to Master Serlo's very conventional, even self-centered, medical career. Indeed, this man is the least reputable of all the court physicians. Master Serlo of Arundel stood a bit apart from the other royal attendants in other ways, too, for he seems to have served Queen Adeliza exclusively. No evidence suggests that he ever treated the king or worked directly with him, although it is possible that he did so. His frequent appearance with the queen in documents suggests that she shared her first husband's delight in associating with medical practitioners. In fact, interest in healing was a family tradition. The king's daughter, Empress Matilda, followed her father in befriending at least one physician; her half-brother, Earl Robert of Gloucester, employed another; and her son, Henry II, would patronize several more.[63]

Serlo was a longtime retainer of Queen Adeliza and frequently attested her charters, almost invariably simply as Master Serlo. The earliest datable mention of him is on the first anniversary of King Henry's death, when he witnessed as Master Serlo, clerk of the queen.[64] He had probably entered her employ some time earlier. Arundel was one of the honors Henry gave his eighteen-year-old bride in 1121, and Serlo may well have been native to this area, where Adeliza later spent much of her time. Many of the queen's clerks were canons of Waltham, so it is equally likely that Serlo had some connection with that Essex house; he certainly knew many of its members.

Only once in the surviving writs did Serlo call himself a physician, and (interestingly) he appeared at that time with another doctor, named Robert.[65] On the other hand, he was most insistent on emphasizing his title, master, which he employed six other times with the widowed queen, once with her brother, Jocelin, twice with Bishop Simon of Worcester, and three times with her second husband, William de Albini Pincerna, earl of Arundel (1140–76).[66]

Nothing significant is known about Serlo's practice beyond his attendance on the queen, but the records reveal his involvement in a couple of shady real estate deals. Whether he chose to deceive, or whether the disturbed wartime conditions caused him to err, he emphatically tried to profit from lands for which he held questionable title. His manipulating was publicly exposed, but that did not prevent him from blandly carrying off the transaction anyway.

The dispute concerned the churches of Berkeley Hernesse in Gloucestershire and eventually involved three important monasteries as well. In 1051 the dissolved Saxon nunnery of Berkeley had been secularized by Earl Godwin, and its jurisdiction over several other churches, the so-called Hernesse, passed to the Berkeley family. During the civil war in the difficult late

1140s, Queen Adeliza somehow came into possession of the Berkeley lordship, and her clerk, Master Serlo, gained the churches. In 1147 or 1148 he wrote to Bishop Simon of Worcester, who was himself a former clerk of the queen, and declared that, with the consent of his lady, Queen Adeliza, he had given Reading Abbey all the churches in the Berkeley Hernesse. However, Serlo also complained that Gloucester Abbey had encroached on his rights over those churches. A cartulary copy of his letter still exists. When Gilbert Foliot, the abbot of Gloucester (1139–48), heard about the proposed transfer, he fired off a strong note to Edward, the abbot of Reading (1136–54). Abbot Gilbert charged that Master Serlo of Arundel — Foliot was the only one to use this apellation — had no legitimate claim to the Berkeley churches and argued that one of his own clerks already held a prebend at Berkeley, which was not subject to Serlo.

Moreover Serlo had asked the monks of Reading for some unspecified compensation for his gift, and Abbot Gilbert tried to prevent Abbot Edward from making such a bargain. He failed. Master Serlo, however, foresaw the prolonged litigation ahead, and he and Reading obtained letters from Queen Adeliza, her husband Earl William, Archbishop Theobald, and Bishop Simon confirming the gift. King Stephen, the Empress Matilda, and Duke Henry Plantagenet also issued charters in Reading's favor, although these documents stress Adeliza's, rather than Serlo's, part. Ultimately Henry II changed his mind about the whole dispute and settled it in favor of Saint Augustine's Bristol and Robert Fitz Harding, the man who had acquired the Berkeley estates.[67]

Such quarrels about land tenure were fairly common in the trying later years of Stephen's reign, but the participants seem to have relished all the legal maneuvering that resulted. Even Adeliza herself attempted to give Reading, the burial place of her royal husband, some dower lands that were not in her power to alienate permanently.[68]

Twice was evidently not enough. In a third, unpleasant instance Adeliza and Earl William deputized Master Serlo and an unsavory character named William Fitz Gervase to demand tribute from certain churches in the diocese of Chichester. Bishop Hilary (1147–69) was forced to order the two men to stop exacting such secular service from ecclesiastical land.[69] The anarchy that permitted these irregularities was hard on many people, yet Serlo pragmatically allowed his talents to serve personal ambitions rather than pressing medical needs.

The last royal physician, Pedro Alfonso, was more altruistic. He was also quite unusual — a convert from Judaism, a visitor from Spain, a student of Islamic scholarship, a famous author, and a dedicated scientist. He roused strong feelings in his contemporaries, fathered a whole generation of active disciples, and, through his many books, influenced countless Europeans in astronomy, mathematics, theology, literature, and medicine.[70]

On June 29, 1109, at the mature age of forty-four, Pedro Alfonso entered Christian history with dazzling pageantry. Before the courtiers of Aragon assembled for the feast of Saints Peter and Paul, he renounced his ancestral Jewish faith and his given name, Moses, and received baptism from Bishop Stephen of Huesca. Standing by as godfather was King Alfonso I (reigned 1102–34), the mighty warrior nicknamed "The Battler." The new Christian took the name Peter, in memory of the saint, and, to honor his royal patron who introduced him to the "springs of heaven" Pedro was also called "son of Alfonso."[71]

Pedro Alfonso, more properly Petrus Alphonsi, had been an important intellectual leader in his own community, a preacher in the synagogue as well as a practicing physician. Since childhood he had witnessed the tumultuous early reconquest of Moslem Spain, the heroic era of El Cid. Now he, too, joined the crusade, but with weapons of pen, parchment, and contemporary learning.

Baptism changed his life. It was is if all his earlier experience and study had been in preparation for a special mission. Somewhat like that earlier convert, Constantine the African, Pedro decided to devote himself to introducing fellow Christians to the accumulated wisdom of the East. However, whereas Constantine had concentrated on translating classical medical texts, the son of Alfonso chose to explore many areas of oriental culture.

First he explained to Jewish friends why he had become a Christian. He then edited humorous folktales and didactic moral lessons. Finally he summarized major works of Islamic science. In every case Pedro examined both the subject itself and how it affected the physiological and psychological life of human beings. Despite time-consuming foreign travel, he carried through this impressive program with astonishing speed and genial good will. Much of his creative outburst occurred while he was in England as personal physician to King Henry and as teacher to several naturalists in the Severn Valley. By 1121 he had returned to Aragon. His literary explosion thus covered less than fifteen years, from 1106 to 1121.

Pedro composed at least eight treatises, six of which are extant in one form or another. They follow in rough chronological order.

1. *Dialogue with a Jew*, sometimes called the *Conversations of Petrus Alphonsi*—a polemical tract justifying Pedro's conversion, probably written shortly after 1106. Pedro the Christian debates with Moses, his former Hebraic self, maintaining that Catholicism is inherently superior to Judaic and Islamic life. The author frequently digresses into natural science and is especially interested in the problem of determining longitude and the affect of climate on human life. There is also a valuable, unbiased discussion of Mohammed. By medieval standards of manuscript distribution the *Dialogue* was a runaway best seller; several twelfth-century English copies still exist. The library at Reading Abbey even had two, one of which was bound with a bestiary.[72]

2. *The Scholar's Guide (Disciplina Clericalis)* — a collection of wry parables and rules of good conduct, probably an early work. Pedro modeled his funny anecdotes of lusty animals, scheming women, and misguided travelers on Arabic stories, which are themselves derived from Jewish, Persian, and Hindu sources, such as Sinbad the Sailor. His edition follows the dialogue format, and first introduced these tales to western readers. It was immensely popular and influenced later writers such as Boccaccio, Chaucer, and Shakespeare. As befits a book of entertainment, there is little medical lore in the *Guide*, but the master does lecture his disciple on the value of good hygiene and of moderation in diet. Medicine is listed among the liberal arts in the place usually reserved for rhetoric. In other allusions, magic is disparaged, and counselors are urged not to stay long in a king's service.[73]

3. *The Tables of al-Khwarizimi* — a series of celestial and calendric computations based on the work of an eminent ninth-century Baghdad astronomer. Pedro constantly refers to a base date of October 1, 1116, which is presumably about the time he composed his study. It is an unsatisfactory adaptation, riddled with errors and reflecting Pedro's distance from his full library. Even contemporary readers annotated its mistakes. Despite such shortcomings, the book was a revelation to western astronomers, like Walcher of Malvern, the first European known to possess an astrolabe. Several different versions appeared, including one by the celebrated Adelard of Bath.[74]

4. *The Dragon* — another astronomical treatise, a complex discussion of the orbital paths of the ascent and descent of the moon. Pedro's own composition is lost, but in 1120 his disciple Walcher wrote out a summary analysis with his master's help. Walcher poignantly reports how sad Master Pedro was that he could not answer every question, having left so many books across the sea.[75]

5. *Letter on Study* — the preface to another lost work of astronomy. This essay exists in both long and short versions (the brief one preceded the al-Khwarizimi astronomical tables) and is a rather preachy, uncharacteristically critical exhortation adressed to French scholars. In it, Pedro indicates that he once gave formal classes to Latin students. Medicine is defined as a "science that guards people's health and is occupied in estimating the length of people's lives in the world." He thus notes the special role of astronomy in therapeutics: it determines the best time for cauterizing, lancing abscesses, bleeding, placing the cupping glass, and tracing fevers. He notes that the books translated by Constantine the African had already demonstrated that astronomy could do such things. Pedro relates the four traditional elements to the changing seasons and to all biological life. He has a sophisticated view of the predictive values of astrology, and he extolls experiment. By this he does not mean the controlled test of an hypothesis, but rather, authentic experience, critical observation, and careful record. Above all, he urges scholars to free themselves from servitude to classical authorities, to study oriental texts, and to use their own faculties.[76]

6. *Parabolae* — a compendium of short maxims from such ancient authors as Cato and Caesar. This undistinguished work is a sober, realistic counterpart to Pedro's delightful *Scholar's Guide*. Doctor Herbert of Durham purchased a copy before 1153.[77]

7. *Humanum Proficium* — a lost booklet that evidently deals with materials from the pseudo-Aristotelian *Secret of Secrets*. Ideas from this famous work were also used in the *Scholar's Guide*. Doctor Herbert owned a copy of part of the *Secret*, but his excerpts could easily have come from the more popular selection John of Seville, made in Spain before 1130, rather than from Pedro's edition.[78]

8. *De Machometo* — another lost work that supposedly discusses the mythical wonders of the East. Pedro may also have composed a treatise on the chronology of different nations.[79]

Throughout these books Pedro appears as a superb teacher — defending his personal choices, disguising hard lessons with jokes, digesting highly technical material, demanding full attention for a new discipline, and demonstrating the relationship of theoretical knowledge to practical therapy. Naturally, the genuine literary and substantive excellence of the books contributed to their success, but they also benefited from the demands of a unique moment in European intellectual history. Christendom was just awakening to the vast traditions of the Arabic, Byzantine, and Jewish worlds and, through them, to a fuller appreciation of classical Greek and Latin thought. Pedro's unusual experience, linguistic skill, and insistent desire to instruct others made him an outstanding pioneer in transmitting this learning to the Christian West.

Within England he also served to link together the royal court, the medical fraternity, and the research community. Walcher of Malvern happily praised Pedro's guidance, and Herbert of Durham was proud to obtain one of his least important books. Adelard of Bath was less generous in acknowledging any mentor, but the evidence — the backdating of most of Adelard's works, the crucial change in his thought about 1115, the similarity of his and Pedro's astronomical studies; and their shared scorn of uncritical reliance upon authority — place him securely within the orbit of the Spaniard's influence. The wide dissemination of Pedro's books to monasteries in Reading, Winchester, Durham, Saint Albans, Worcester, and Canterbury further graphs the extent of his affect.[80]

The situation at Worcester is particularly interesting. On Saturday, December 8, 1128, John, the chronicler of the abbey, observed a series of unusual brilliant sunspots. Shortly thereafter he made a simplified symmetrical drawing to record the rare phenomenon. About the same time, he transcribed Walcher's two treatises and Adelard's al-Khwarizimi tables in another manuscript, and to them he added a sketch of an astrolabe plotted for a latitude close to Worcester and a concordance for the solar eclipse of

August 2, 1133. In 1138 John praised the astronomical tables and, probably to show that he understood them, offered a similar concordance for that year. This is the same author, incidentally, who recorded and illustrated Grimbald's account of King Henry's nightmares.[81]

The connection between Malvern and Worcester was not purely accidental, for a bond of confraternity had existed between the two monasteries well before 1125, probably even before 1117. One of John's other associates was William of Malmesbury, the best informed, most tolerant writer about Islam during a period when most people enjoyed only silly tales about Mohammed. Perhaps he was another of Pedro's contacts; they certainly had a common interest in medicine.[82]

Unlike other royal physicians, Pedro does not appear in nonliterary records. He did not attest any known mandates of either King Alfonso or King Henry, an odd situation considering his wide reputation and his persistent feeling of self-importance. Fortunately, his personal preambles contain the forms of his name and snatches of biography. The account of his baptism, for example, was incorporated in the preface to the *Dialogue*, and the fact that he was King Henry's physician was preserved at the beginning of a copy of the *Scholar's Guide*.[83]

Besides his books, Pedro created a second legacy. Within his lifetime, and perhaps inspired by his teaching, a remarkable exodus of brilliant young Englishmen crossed to Spain to study classical and oriental science and to translate Islamic and Hebraic tomes into Latin. The greatest names in this parade—Daniel of Morley, Alfred of Sareshel, Roger of Hereford, and Alexander Neckam—belong to the last quarter of the century, but the two Britons, William and Glaucus, were working with John of Seville long before 1150.

An even more important transitional figure and possible protegé of Pedro Alfonso is Robert of Ketton, who can be found in Toledo as early as 1141. His birthplace was evidently Ketton, in tiny Rutland, but he was sometimes also called Robert of Chester. He returned to London by 1147 and, like so many medieval scientists, prepared his own study of the astrolabe. Several of his other treatises were actually revisions of Adelard of Bath's works, such as a new version of the troublesome al-Khwarizimi tables and a revised *Mappae Clavicula*, or manual of chemical formulas. Robert and Pedro have not yet been connected, but both were active in the same area of Spain, and the old master would have been pleased that this Englishman, at least, was continuing his own manifold interests.[84]

Pedro Alfonso was in his late fifties when he left England, and it is unlikely that he ever returned. In Spain he reappears in connection with two prosaic matters. On April 14, 1121, he attested a bill of sale for a French knight who had just acquired lands in the recently conquered Ebro Valley. He was not given any prominence in the deed, which hardly demonstrates any renewed eminence at court. A final mention in September, 1141, is less reliable. A Pedro Alfos witnessed another property transaction in the same valley, but the cartulary record is confusing. Pedro's name is given in a second list of subscribers to the writ, and the copyist included it within brackets and in a different color ink. If this Pedro is the physician, he would have been about eighty at the time. He had had a great life, and one likes to assume that he ended it with his usual engaging style and good will.[85]

King Henry's eight physicians spotlight the diversity of medical types active in Norman England. John of Tours was a ruthless, self-taught, old-school practitioner, ridiculed by younger men. Ranulf turned from medicine and its financial rewards to monastic contemplation. Clarembald was evidently as concerned about the publication of his research as about actual practice. Nigel of Calne, an early pluralist, submerged his medical skill in his administrative service of king and viceroy. Faritius was a prototype of innumerable later doctors, who enriched themselves and enlarged their charities as much through soothing demeanor as through authentic craft. Grimbald was a tireless family physician, forever traveling about, even making house calls in the dead of night. He was a faithful companion, doting father, occasional dream interpreter, and garrulous raconteur. Master Serlo of Arundel chose a smaller compass for his life, serving few people and missing no opportunity to extend his own influence. Pedro Alfonso was the bridge to the wider worlds of science and literature, and of Jewish and Islamic scholarship.

These physicians were bookish men who took intellectual matters seriously. Yet their collections of relics, miracles, and marvels implied no contradiction of their expertise. Although not accepting of every strange tale, they felt no need to be skeptical about inexplicable events. Not all wonders were analyzed with microscopic detachment; miracles could be viewed as suspensions of natural law, but they were also normal parts of life, indications of the power of divine grace operating in the world. It was judged miraculous if a blind man gained sight, if a particularly difficult wound healed, if a poet created a splendid song, if a sinner repented—the wonder was less in the act than in the prior intention of the suppliant.

Such attitudes help to explain why an intellectually curious ruler like Henry welcomed the companionship of physicians. These healers always retained something of their mystery. The Normans had a passion for organization, but when a detailed analysis of King Henry's household, the so-called *Constitutio Domus Regis*, was drawn up late in the reign, physicians were not included. Apparently they maintained a special relationship with the king. Rather than receive a fixed salary like other retainers, they directly sought their duties and rewards at his pleasure. On the other hand, the lives of the practitioners did not revolve about the king alone. To these complex individuals, with independent, satisfying interests all their own, royal service was the dominant, but not the only, concern.

Although they could be vain, ambitious, and greedy, Anglo-Norman physicians were far from being despised or ineffective. The known royal practitioners and probably most of their hundreds of silent colleagues appear to have been worthy servants of a demanding profession, nobly striving to alleviate human suffering. To judge from the testimony of persistent crown interest, broad-based community support, and generous ecclesiastical assistance, their contemporaries appreciated their efforts.

IV. THE RISE OF
INSTITUTIONAL CARE

Early twelfth-century people were unusually creative individuals. Their sparkling developments in ecclesiastical architecture, manuscript illumination, university education, scholastic philosophy, and romantic poetry enlarged the lives of generations to come. England's special contributions to such progress were often pragmatic, rather than aesthetic or intellectual. The country's leaders and subjects enthusiastically embraced challenges in governmental administration, labor-saving technology, and public welfare. Their concern promoted innovative changes in areas such as jury justice, exchequer finance, mechanical power, and, especially, community-based health care.

Indeed, the new hospitals were a principal way in which the century's highest ideals achieved concrete reality. These institutions ranged from tiny shelters for handfuls of members to multidepartmental complexes with hundreds of bed patients. The term hospital itself was vital and flexible; encompassing hostels for travelers and indigent students, dispensaries for poor relief, clinics and surgeries for the injured, homes for the blind, the lame, the elderly, the orphaned, and the mentally ill, and leprosaria for people of all ages and classes. A single unit frequently combined many of these functions. Most facilities, however, probably resembled modern nursing homes, for custodial care and rehabilitation therapy were particularly emphasized.[1]

Love of God, compassion for humanity, and concern for their own welfare encouraged people to build hospitals. Almost half were directly affiliated with monasteries, priories, and churches. Many hospitals, imitating religious communities, formulated precise rules of conduct, required a uniform type of dress, and integrated several worship services into their daily routine. However, the traditional spiritual context of the hospitals enhanced, but did not overshadow, their genuine therapeutic achievements.

The practice of nursing sick relatives, friends, and allies must be as old as time itself, but the momentous breakthrough to institutional care only came within the reach of most people early in the twelfth century. Unfortunately, few later commentators appreciated this development. In fact, it has long been fashionable to claim that early medieval facilities were not yet "true" hospitals, that is, professional centers with physicians, laboratories, medicines, operations, and convalescing patients. Even so gracious an authority as Rotha Mary Clay underestimated the healing mission of the medieval hospital by declaring that it was "an ecclesiastical not a medical institution." Others gave credit for the rise of "true" hospitals in western Europe to the crusaders, especially the Hospitaller Knights of Saint John, who supposedly brought back improved medical concepts from Byzantium and the Levant.[2] Despite frequent repetition of these assertions, none now seems tenable, at least for Britain.

Despite the near-absence of details of patient care and the infrequent references to surgical operations, it is clear that the Anglo-Norman hospital rose from a drive to alleviate human suffering as well as from a desire to assist people to understand their lot in life. Founders, benefactors, and staff officers endeavored to help the sick and not merely house them, and that is exactly what they did. The clearest proof of their success is the widespread popular support their hospitals immediately attracted. The continuing demand for additional facilities was never satisfied.

The sheer numbers of English institutions called hospitals are extremely impressive, and form the larger context for any valid discussion of institutional purpose and routine. Much later, in the fourteenth century, the national statistics would crest at about 700 individual hospitals, but the first waves were even more significant. The original tidal surge is beyond sight, but the depths of its successors can be estimated.

7	hospitals before 1066
14	more between 1066 and 1100
92	more between 1100 and 1154
113	cumulative total in 1154

Moreover, these figures represent only a fraction of the actual facilities, including neither the well-designed monastic infirmaries, nor the preceptories of the crusading Hospitallers, nor the small communities of nuns who attended the sick. Many tiny hospitals never entered the records at all. On the other hand, at least 33 additional hospitals were founded at undetermined periods within the twelfth century, but cannot yet be securely placed before 1154.

Of course, the foundation dates of hospitals, or of any medieval institution, cannot be too precise because the establishment of a house was a complex and lengthy process. A date could mean the moment a founder first declared his intention, or the time of his first endowment, or the year the site was occupied, or the day completed buildings were finally blessed. Decades might intervene between any one of these stages. At the other end of the scale, some hospitals ceased to exist entirely, while others were simply refounded under new names.

King Henry's own hospital foundations demonstrate the authentic concern for public health already glimpsed in his association with physicians, as well as in his curiosity about marvels and his increasing concept of social responsibility. Dozens of additional facilities were established by Henry's barons and retainers and, above all, by the church leaders of his time — certainly the most imaginative providers of health care. However, a significant portion of hospital development was also the direct result of local community action, of average people improving their own lives.

All these efforts were the outgrowth of a heritage centuries old. The legions of Roman Britain had devised a carefully organized system of military medicine, which included a common structural design of sick wards around an open courtyard. Remains of about twenty-five such complexes can be identified, mostly strung along the northern frontier. About A.D. 85 one hospital compound at Inchtuthil, in Scotland, had sixty-four wards and was capable of treating more than 250 soldiers simultaneously. By Norman times these sturdy halls were only buried ruins, and no Roman influence is detectable on medieval models. One twelfth-century facility was, however, built within the shell of a Roman bath.[3]

The Venerable Bede mentioned a hospital, and certain place names in Wales suggest the existence of several more, but the first enduring foundations and the initial flower of royal concern seem to have occurred under Athelestan, the earliest true king of all England (reigned 924–40).[4] Support came from clerics and nobles, as well as from the court. For example, about 927 a pilgrim named Guy of Warwick stopped at a small hospital in Winchester called Saint Cross. This may have been erected by the monk, Saint Brinstan, who was bishop of Winchester from 931 to 934. Evidently it later came to be identified with Saint John's Hospital in the High Street. In the north, a hospital at Flixton, in eastern Yorkshire, claimed that its founder was Acehorne, a thane of King Athelestan. His house was intended to maintain fourteen men and women and to protect travelers from wild beasts.

The king's own foundation, Saint Peter's Hospital in the city of York, was begun in 937 after Athelestan's triumphant return from defeating the Scots and Norse at the battle of Brunanburh. The campaign had devastated the area, and the king, taking pity on some refugees, granted them the princely endowment called Petercorn. This meant that his new foundation was entitled to collect a *thrave* (a certain number of sheaves of wheat) from each *caracuate* (a unit of land capable of supporting one family for one year) ploughed in the district. It was quite a heavy tax, and consequently Saint Peter's became a mighty institution, the largest hospital in all Britain. Needless to say, its governors always cultivated a special relationship with succeeding monarchs.

Athelestan also patronized other charities. He ordered that alms be given regularly to the poor and leprous of Bath, and his descendants continued this stipend. He endowed northern minsters such as Beverley and Ripon and funded their libraries. It is probably no coincidence that at about this time the major monument of Saxon medicine, Bald's *Leechbook*, was compiled. Athelestan's own inspiration may have been due in part to his friendship with the Welsh King Hwyel Dda of Dyfed (910–40), who had a very high regard for physicians, giving them precedence at his court and mentioning them in his legal codes.[5] Thus, Athelestan's era marks something of a hopeful dawn in English health care. Full daylight was long delayed, however.

Despite the promising start in the early tenth century, only four other hospitals can be identified for the remaining pre-Conquest years.[6] The blaze came with the Normans. With characteristic gusto these brash warriors set about erecting medical facilities shortly after subjugating the country. Sumptuous Battle Abbey was built on the very spot of William's victory at Hastings. Sometime before 1076 a hospital, or at least a hospice for pilgrims and travelers, was erected outside its main gate. The Conqueror also endowed a leper hospital at Northampton. The most important medical leadership for the kingdom, however, came from Archbishop Lanfranc of Canterbury. Beginning about 1080–84 he erected in rapid succession Saint John's Hospital at the Northgate of Canterbury, Saint Gregory's Hospital right across the street, and Saint Nicholas's Hospital at Harbledown about a mile beyond the Westgate.

Saint John's was for the aged, the poor, and the sick, and housed about one hundred men and women. It was an impressive sight and the chronicler Eadmer praised its great stone buildings.[7] Appearances have changed over the centuries, but Saint John's still functions as a retirement home. It may well be the oldest almshouse in Britain still doing the work for which it was intended. Originally it consisted of a large hall, chapel, and several other buildings around a large courtyard. Eadmer said that one part was for women, the other for men. The main hall had semicircular arches and doorways and was shaped like a capital letter *T*, or a Tau cross, with the chapel in the post arm and the residents in the lintel. The light-colored walls of this structure, once perhaps two stories high, still stand open to the sky beyond the present chapel, which has a transplanted Norman door. Saint John's was endowed with extensive suburban property, part of which is now the campus of the University of Kent.

Nearby Saint Gregory's began as a hospital, but it quickly became a home for aged priests and for clergy working at Saint John's.[8] Saint Gregory's evidently began with six priests, who were to tend the sick across the street. Each priest had two clerks to assist him, and they were all to live in common. Lanfranc seems to have used this hospital as a catch-all for his diocesan charities, and it may have even taken up much of the pastoral work of the cathedral. The archbishop certainly placed the grammar and music schools of the town under its direction.[9] To carry on these works Lanfranc handsomely endowed the hospital with the tithes of some area churches and with other privileges. Domesday Book further indicates that the young hospital owned thirty-two houses and a mill in the town and had twelve tenants paying rent. The eighteen men on the staff and their uncounted servants were certainly not overburdened by the schoolboys, aged priests, and hundred-odd patients at Saint John's. However, financial independence and light duties did not prevent the so-called hospital from becoming involved in unedifying quarrels with Saint Augustine's Abbey over the reburial of certain Saxon saints.

Very early in the episcopate of Archbishop William of Corbeil (1123–36), Saint Gregory's ceased to offer independent medical service and became strictly a priory of thirteen canons under the newly introduced rule of Saint Augustine. Undoubtedly the Austins continued to perform some work for Saint John's but not to the extent of the previous commitment. The history of Saint Gregory's illustrates several contemporary practices: the brief span of some hospitals; their intimate connection with education; the rivalry of all institutions for prestige and privilege; the temptation to direct greater resources to administrators than to patients; and the program of replacing secular clergy with formally organized religious, usually regular canons. The civic-minded Austin canons staffed many hospitals in their early fervent days, but, as the decades slipped by, they converted several of the institutions to their private conventual use. Thus, after closing as a hospital, Saint Gregory's remained a small priory until its dissolution under Henry VIII.

On a wooded hill overlooking the city, Saint Nicholas Harbledown enjoyed a better history of community service and, like Saint John's Northgate, still continues the good work today. Lanfranc had planned a surprisingly large hospital for thirty male and thirty female lepers, but it soon grew to a full hundred, and the residents must have been uncomfortably crowded on the small, steeply sloped hillside. The archbishop ordered that the lepers be cared for by a chaplain and skillful, patient, and kindly watchers. Apparently the patients were thought to need fewer priests than the folk at Saint John's, perhaps because there was no school at Harbledown.

The hill was crowned by a plain romanesque church with a round apse, extensively enlarged in the early twelfth century, maybe due to the increased population. The present structure still incorporates in its fabric several features of this Norman rebuilding—the round arches and strong pillars of the north side of the nave, the square tower, and the western door. Interestingly, the floor of the church gently slopes away from the altar, perhaps to allow more efficient disinfection and cleansing with water. As late as 1815 a thirteenth-century screen still bisected the nave from east to west, separating the brothers and sisters.

Outside, medieval residents apparently lived in wooden huts scattered about the hill. Communal buildings, including a great hall, probably underlie the present accommodations. In King Henry I's time Saint Nicholas was called the Hospital of the Wood of Blean. Its prosperity and fame increased over the years. Henry himself allowed the lepers to increase their acreage by clearing away ten perches (165 feet) of thicket from the perimeter of the hospital.[10] His grandson, Henry II, did penance there after the murder of Thomas Becket and gave the inmates a yearly stipend. Many people, including the afflicted Black Prince (d. 1376) thought its spring water had special medicinal qualities.

Lanfranc was probably concentrating on Canterbury's own residents, rather than on the town's growing number of pilgrims, when he created such multiple hospital facilities. As archbishop he was very conscious of his local community responsibilities. His monastic constitutions provided that an almoner from the abbey should visit the sick and do good works about the town. He even attempted to regulate commerce by establishing a standard liquid measure; in fact, a century later a daily ration of beer was still reckoned as "Lanfranc's measure."[11] The inspiration for his civic concern was probably rooted in his own personality, learning, and Italian upbringing, but his monastic cathedral chapter did include a couple of distinguished physicians who may have urged him to open public hospitals.

Oddly, neither William Rufus nor Archbishop Anselm seems to have championed the burgeoning hospital movement. Rufus did, however, arrange for the transfer of Saint Peter's York to a new location not far from its old site. On the other hand, Lanfranc's legacy visibly excited King Henry and his wives and his associates. The pace of hospital construction dramatically accelerated early in his reign and never slackened thereafter. In fact, an average of two hospitals opened each year between 1100 and 1154, in good times and bad. Considering that the national population was only about two million and that many larger building programs were competing for attention and funding, this is a very remarkable record.

Like the physicians, the hospitals blanketed the map of the kingdom, although not in quite the same distribution. Thirty-two different counties gained hospitals in 1154. As befits its premier size, Yorkshire had the greatest number of facilities (fifteen), but small, wealthy, heavily populated Norfolk was second with fourteen. As expected, certain shires with major urban concentrations were well served—Kent (seven), Hampshire (six), and Middlesex (six)—but so was Sussex (seven), a more rural area. At least twenty towns could boast of two or more hospitals, yet there were also striking omissions. No early hospice has so far come to light in Bristol or Salisbury (Old Sarum), or in such counties as Bedford, Dorset, Lancashire, and Surrey.

One barometer of the movement is the surprising ratio of individual places to total population. In effect, at least one hospital bed was available for every 1,000 persons; there may even have been one for every 600 persons, a very favorable proportion by any standard.

Briefly, the ratio was estimated in the following way.

  861   known beds from 32 hospitals
1,053   estimated beds (81 other hospitals x 13, the most frequent unit size)

1,914   total beds
2,000,000 people ÷ 1,914 × 1,044.93, or a ratio 1:1,000

This estimate could be refined in several ways. For example,
  861   known beds
2,187   (81 × 27 [the average size hospital, 861 ÷ 32])
  446   (27 × 16 [half of 33 undatable twelfth-century hospitals])

3,494   total beds
2,000,000 ÷ 3,494 × 572, or a ratio 1:572

Every medieval statistic is somewhat artificial, but, because of lost information, these approximations probably underestimate the twelfth-century reality, Nevertheless, the perception that there was one hospital bed for every 600 to 1,000 persons can be a useful gauge of early care. As with the physicians, Norman England seems to have been better served by hospitals than was France at the same time. In absolute numbers there were more French facilities, but they covered a larger area and population. Modern figures offer further insight. In England today the ratio of hospital beds to citizens is 1:108; in the United States it is 1:227.[12] Granted, there are indeed substantial differences in these calculations. Current totals, for example, do not count retirement and nursing home residents. On the other hand, whereas modern people demand endless, often unnecessary, professional service, the Anglo-Normans treated a far larger share of health and geriatric problems at home. Thus the need for beds was not regarded as important in the middle ages as it is today, rendering this ratio all the more significant.

It is interesting that some English towns boast ratios spectacularly better than any of these figures. For example, the quite solid information for Winchester reveals that in 1148 the town had six hospitals and a reliably estimated population of eight thousand. Three of the hospitals had a known capacity of fifty-two beds and thirty-nine more can be guessed for the other three. Thus in Winchester there was one bed available to every ninety burghers. In Canterbury the ratio would have even been better, but, of course, the town attracted the sick from a much wider area.

How did such a sudden proliferation of Norman hospitals come about? No thundering preacher or brilliant publicist popularized the new social gospel, and few causal relationships can be detected among the institutions themselves. The answer seems to be that, working cooperatively but without self-conscious unity, four groups—the royal family, the clergy, barons, and average citizens—all decided it was to their advantage to build hospitals. Thus the ninety-three facilities created between 1100 and 1154 could list as known patrons: one king, three queens, eleven bishops, nine religious superiors, eleven major barons, four noble women, twenty less important persons ranging from monks to courtiers to townsfolk.

Many other individuals, especially women, offered additional subsidiary support. Compassionate charity, private penance, family prestige, and community need were all motivating factors, but most donors concentrated on quite local problems rather than developing any theory of comprehensive national health service.

Some shrewd contributors considered their gifts to be insurance policies that would eventually pay dividends. Such patrons primarily aided hospitals in order to insure future places for the sick and the aged members of their own families or religious communities. In time, the houses that accepted such qualified gifts often turned into retirement homes, not for the poor, but for "distressed gentlefolk."

Most philanthropists were more altruistic. Sincerely distressed by the sight of others less fortunate, they specifically reserved their foundations for the poor, the infirm, or the sick poor. Consequently it is sometimes difficult to separate health care from relief for the poor. Outright almshouses and the hospices for indigent pilgrims both had a fairly obvious purpose, but they constituted only a fraction of the new institutions. On the other hand, hospitals were frequently built at river crossings and not only had responsibilities for wayfarers and the sick, but also for maintaining the local bridges. This is an interesting vestige of the early work of hermits, who had long had similar obligations and who were the first great promoters of hospital care. Above all, however, founders were anxious to help the lepers, and there was no doubt in anyone's mind that these victims were sick and needed specialized attention. Almost half of all the new institutions were specifically designated for those who were thought to have contracted the dread malady.[13]

By any measure, King Henry and his wives were the greatest hospital patrons. They created new institutions, endowed existing houses, and encouraged their vassals to build others. Queen Matilda began the benefactions, and she set the pattern for royal support for the next fifty years. As early as

1101 she decided to sponsor a large leper hospital, Saint Giles-in-the-Fields, at Holborn, just outside the bounds of London. Her gift may have been related to what seems to have been a difficult first pregnancy. The works of Archbishop Lanfranc also probably inspired her, but the greatest influence may have been that of her mother, saintly Margaret of Scotland. Like Matilda, Margaret loved the arts and learning and built a hospital at Edinburgh dedicated to Saint Giles (d. c. 710), a hermit protector of cripples, lepers, and nursing mothers. Incidentally, Queen Margaret had frequently corresponded with Lanfranc, so a Canterbury connection is probably in the background, after all.

In the London area, besides Saint Giles, there was a second nearby leper hospital, Saint James, in Westminster; but whether it predates or succeeds Matilda's foundation is still uncertain. Witnesses testified that it had been established by the citizens of London earlier than anyone could remember. Matilda's daughter had a special devotion to the apostle James the Greater, and King Henry obtained a major relic of the martyr for his abbey at Reading, so it is possible that this Westminster hospital may have been another of the queen's good works. Saint James was designed to treat fourteen leprous maidens. The fact that it was planned for young girls is of special interest because children constitute the group most highly susceptible to leprosy.

Queen Matilda was famous, even notorious, for her devotion to the lepers. She apparently brought them right into her own chamber in the palace of Westminster, fed them, and in Biblical fashion washed their feet. On one of these occasions her brother David found her in the midst of such ablutions and gave her a stern rebuke. King Henry, he felt, would hardly be anxious to kiss her once he had learned that she caressed the feet of such people so ardently. David was quite devout himself, and later as king of Scotland he founded numerous religious houses of all types. Matilda evidently had considerable influence on the young prince for in this instance she soon prevailed on him also to kiss the lepers. The episode, probably recounted by David, impressed a number of later writers, but particularly Robert of Gloucester, a thirteenth-century chronicler, who was Matilda's chief panegyrist. He claimed that her various charities were responsible for introducing a new, enlightened attitude toward lepers in England.[14]

By medieval standards Matilda's hospital of Saint Giles was quite large, housing forty patients. Her principal grant was a yearly subsidy of sixty shillings from her wharf at Queenhythe, on the Thames, a stipend that was still being paid four centuries later. The size of her donation accorded well with the tight-fisted finance of her husband and with the realization that a founder's protection, prestige, and fund raising potential were often the most valuable contributions. As expected, her example inspired other gifts. One subject, Robert Fitz Ralph, who may have been a leper himself, gave so much that some people thought of him as the founder. In fact, once having

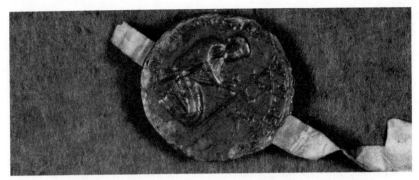

WALTER, PRIOR OF SAINT JOHN'S HOSPITAL

About 1148 Walter, the English master of the Hospitaller Knights and prior of their facility at Saint John's Clerkenwell, ended a dispute with the nearby nuns of Saint Mary's Convent. On the seal attached to his writ he is shown kneeling before a patriarchial cross. By permission of the British Library, Harley Charter 83 C 40.

begun the hospital and having granted it a yearly dividend, Matilda cleverly made the citizens of London responsible for further upkeep. One of her chaplains, a man named John, was probably the first master; mention is made of him in 1118. Hospital administrators were not usually physicians, but it is worth recalling that a John medicus held land in London in 1128x1138. He was probably a layman, however.[15]

Queen Matilda's creation of Saint Giles-in-the-Fields probably had a political dimension, too. In 1101 Henry was still regarded as a usurper king and was being challenged for England's throne by his foolish older brother, Robert Curthose of Normandy. London, the greatest city of Henry's kingdom, was overwhelmingly Saxon in population and local leadership. Matilda, the descendant of Saxon kings, could easily have been bidding for the city's continued allegiance by endowing an impressive, badly needed facility designed to treat London's most serious health problem.[16]

Before her death in 1118 Matilda founded a second, or third, leprosarium, this one at Chichester. It was a small house built for a master or chaplain and eight leprous brothers and was dedicated to Saints James and Mary Magdalene. Although the queen devoted considerable personal energies to these hospitals and undoubtedly had the support of her husband in granting their lands and rents, no special privileges of confirmations for them from the king himself have yet appeared in the records.

It would be wrong, however, to think that Henry left all charitable enterprise to his wife, or that his own concern and political sensitivity surfaced only after his son's tragic death in 1120. For example, in the countryside of northern Yorkshire, far from London's problems, Goathland typifies the nature of Henry's early involvement. The poor in that remote area were attracted to a priest named Osmund, who was living as a hermit. Disciples as well as dependents came, and soon an informal community offered varied assistance, including health care, to those in need. Within a short time the hospice came to the king's attention, perhaps because it was occupying royal land. From his court at Windsor Henry issued a writ granting Osmund and his brethern land at Goathland to maintain the poor, stating that they should enjoy his peace. This last remark was a significant concession and was partially directed to the royal foresters, who were thereby ordered not to disturb the group.

Sometime later the king visited the city of York and heard more about Osmund's work. Thereupon he increased the community's endowment by adding a modest amount of acreage for ploughing and some pastureland for herds. As responsibilities and membership increased, the hermits felt the need to regularize their personal religious situation. With the king's consent, they surrendered their hermitage to the nearby abbey of Whitby, and all took the monastic habit there, sometime before 1114. The good work at Goathland continued but now under the abbey's general supervision.[17]

Notice of this obscure house survived because it later became part of the record of a large monastic corporation. Yet Goathland's microcosmic experience reflects the unheralded relief spontaneously offered in many parts of the kingdom, the unsystematic but not unsympathetic aid of the government, and the increasing institutionalization of all social services.

Whitby Abbey was a vigorous house, only recently reestablished within the ruins of the famous Saxon monastery destroyed by the Danes in 867. During the same time that it was welcoming Goathland, Whitby was creating a second hospital with another hermit. In 1109 a leper named Orm had sought assistance, and Abbot William de Percy had granted him a bit of land that came to be called Spittalbridge, a graphic title similarly applied to many other early leper houses. The monks also provided food, clothing, and the right to be buried in their abbey sanctuary. Soon more lepers and other patients joined Orm, and the loose association became a hospital dedicated to Saint Michael. The new hospital's master, Robert d'Aunay, an aristocrat-turned-hermit asked help from a wealthy relation, Gundreda de Gournay.

Gundreda was a logical choice for her family was intimately connected with Whitby. Her late husband, Nigel d'Aubigny, had been one of the barons specifically charged by the king to protect Goathland. Moreover, when Nigel became gravely ill at Durham a short time later (1109x1114) he tried to make his peace with God by restoring lands he had taken from all sorts of institutions, including Saint Peter's Hospital in York and Whitby Abbey. This contrition was evidently successful for Nigel recovered, and later he and Gundreda had a son, Roger de Mowbray, who grew up to be a notable patron of monasteries and hospitals, especially Burton Lazars in Leicester.[18]

In 1130x1138 when she was approached by Robert d'Aunay, Gundreda probably thought of Whitby with mixed feelings. Therefore she gave Saint Michael's leper hospital at Spittalbridge only a couple of plots of land, worth an annual rent of six shillings.[19] She had become caught up in the hospital movement, however, and shortly thereafter gave Saint Peter's York several plots at Bagby, in north Yorkshire. Her charter does not actually declare that she wished to found a hospital there, but this must have been the understanding because such a facility for the poor and the sick, locally called "Spital," was built shortly thereafter. Paulinus, the doctor of York, was one of the witnesses to Gundreda's grant, and a Master Berner, perhaps Bernard, the medicus of Durham and York, attested her son's deed of confirmation a few years later. Paulinus is particularly interesting as one of the few Anglo-Norman physicians associated with a hospital. Perhaps Paulinus was the go-between in establishing Bagby as a satellite of Saint Peter's, another unusual development in an era when most hospitals were separate from one another.[20]

At Whitby Abbot Bernard (c. 1139–48) thought that one of his monks, Geoffrey Mansall, had contracted leprosy and sent him to live at Spittalbridge. This soon became the normal practice. The abbey made ample provisions for inmates at Saint Michael's, giving each person a weekly ration of bread and beer and a daily main meal of fish or meat, similar to that in the convent itself.[21] King Henry did not specifically help this leper hospital or the newer house at Bagby, but on more than one occasion he did grant the abbey full confirmation of its many privileges.[22] He was even more directly generous to the large hospital of Saint Peter, which was traditionally the beneficiary of great royal favors. To emphasize his connection with this famous old center, Henry would describe himself as its protector and brother when making a gift. Stephen later used a similar phrase.[23]

The Goathland hospital was an early example of King Henry's interest in social welfare, but it was never a major institution. Far more significant in terms of numbers of people treated and general influence on the quality of life were the several leper hospitals the king founded in urban centers: Saint Bartholomew in Oxford; Saint James in Bridgenorth; Saint Giles in Shrewsbury; Saint Mary Magdalene in Newcastle. Another royal foundation, Saint John the Evangelist in Cirencester, a much smaller town, was attached to the monastery of Austin canons, which Henry founded in 1117 and raised to a full abbey in 1131. It was intended for the poor of the area.

Queen Adeliza, Henry's second wife, also founded hospitals. At Wilton she built Saint Giles, a lazar house, and later, after she was widowed, she endowed a small pilgrim hospice at Pynham, in Sussex. Like many hospitals this was built near a bridge and the canons had special additional obligations to keep the causeway open.[24] In 1148 Stephen's queen, Matilda, founded the hospital of Saint Katherine, next to the Tower of London, for thirteen lepers.[25] The foundations of King Henry and the three queens, Matilda, Adeliza, and Matilda, account for more than ten percent of the new hospitals in the country.

The support roll was longer yet, however, for Henry was instrumental in setting up additional urban leper facilities such as Holy Innocents, Lincoln—where he was said to be the founder, although the house may have been established by Bishop Remigius (d. 1092)—and such as Saint Mary Magdalene, Colchester, and Saint Mary Magdalene, Reading. The Colchester experience suggests something of how the king's mind worked, how he enlisted governmental officials to share his charities, and how he cautiously moved from quite specific targets to larger objectives. In 1096 Eudo, the seneschal of William Rufus, founded the abbey of Saint John, Colchester. In the new reign he happily served Henry and steadily gained prizes for his monastery, including in 1102 a modest hunting privilege "for the work of the monks' infirmary." Later, at Henry's insistence, he and the monks moved beyond convent concerns and set up the leper hospital of Saint Mary. After Eudo's death in 1120, Henry fleetingly considered marrying the seneschal's widow, Rose, but he chose Adeliza of Louvain instead. He maintained his interest in Colchester largely by reconfirming some of Eudo's earlier donations. One royal writ insured that the hospital would receive at least six pounds a year from some of the steward's properties.[26] Henry was wise to separate the hospital's endowments from those of the abbey. Later, hospital residents claimed he had given them additional perquisites, but, lacking the necessary royal charters to prove their case, they failed to carry the point. They blamed an earlier abbot for burning the lost charters.[27]

Henry may have encouraged a similar expansion from infirmary to hospital facilities at Abingdon. He definitely inspired other royal officials such as the clerks, Richard de Brecon and Thomas, at Saint James Bridgenorth, and helped his courtier Rahere at Smithfield, outside London. One of the royal chamberlains, Herbert, established a small hospital outside the Westgate of Winchester, but it does not seem to have endured. Nearby, five shacks or cottages were erected for the poor by a certain "Osbert, son of Thiard."[28] These tiny accommodations were probably typical of many small clinics and residences that enjoyed relatively brief lives.

In his own right Henry also gave pastures, ploughland, rents, fairs, daily stipends, water mills, wood for fuel, freedom from tolls, and outright alms to many other institutions. Thus, in addition to aiding Saint Peter's, where the king was traditionally a special patron, Henry significantly endowed the hospitals of Saint Nicholas Harbledown, Saint Paul Norwich, Saint Bartholomew Smithfield, and Saint Bartholomew Rochester.[29] It is interesting that, except for those to the lepers at Harbledown, the gifts were for metropolitan hospitals for the sick. Evidently the king preferred to found leper houses but still felt an obligation to support general service facilities. There were also special alms for the sick at Derby, perhaps a gift to an unidentified hospital there, and general alms in other places.[30] Early gifts to monastic infirmaries sometimed preceded grants to hospitals in the same area, almost as if the king were enlarging his concept of charity.[31] These expenses were all paralleled by his other major gifts to monasteries and churches throughout the country.

Moreover, at the same time he was providing for English needs, Henry was also endowing monasteries and hospitals in his duchy of Normandy. He even helped institutions in France, including the famous leper hospital at Chartres.[32] Frequently, the cash value of these overseas gifts was greater than those he made to insular houses, but they were also less numerous. Perhaps the happiest gift of all came from Henry's daughter, the Empress Matilda; it was one of that haughty woman's few inspired ideas. To commemorate her father's great love for lepers she set up a fund which insured that each year, on the anniversary of his death, a gala banquet was provided for all lepers within reach of York.[33]

King Stephen, on the other hand, was a colorless, unimaginative patron. His best gifts were to Saint Peter's York, which he helped reconstruct after a disastrous fire in 1137, and to Saint Mary Magdalene Colshester. Naturally he cooperated with his wife in establishing Saint Katherine London, but, except for the possibility of one small hospital in Norwich, his writs were merely confirmations of donations previously made by King Henry.[34]

Fortunately, other Norman leaders were more forward-looking. Of the ninety-three hospitals founded between 1100 and 1154, fully 42 percent were directly affiliated with and subordinated to religious communities. Of these, 20 percent were sponsored by monastic congregations. The plan at Abingdon was fairly typical. The hospital (now the town's guildhall) was erected beside the main gate of the abbey, available for the protection and service of the monks but intended for the general public. A further 16 percent of the religiously affiliated hospitals were run by Austin canons or by the uniquely English Gilbertine nuns and canons. Lastly, 6 percent were connected with the hospital and military orders which grew out of the crusades — the Hospitallers of Saint John, the Knights of the Holy Sepulchre, the Templars, and the order of Saint Lazarus of Jerusalem.

The crusading groups were less significant than has often been assumed. Their facilities introduced few new ideas into England and came in the 1140's after the tide of hospital construction had long risen. Moreover, the crusaders' hospitals were primarily intended for each order's own sick and aged members. On the other hand, crusading groups, especially the Hospitallers, were very anxious to train their own men in medicine. Thus Saint John's Hospital in Clerkenwell, the Hospitallers' headquarters, probably came as close to being a formal medical school as any place in Britain.

Hospitals not associated with religious orders were much more autonomous and constituted 58 percent, a clear majority, of the whole. They included major establishments such as Saint Peter's York and Saint Nicholas Harbledown, and quite small transitory facilities like the one built by Herbert the Chamberlain in Winchester.

Faint connections are discernible among a few foundations, like Bagby and York. Such ties often originated from family and friend relationships. For example, about 1125x1135 Bishop Alexander of Lincoln opened a leper hospital, Saint Leonard, at Newark-on-Trent, and used for his model the great hospital of York. He even brought down Robert, the almoner of York, to manage its affairs. Spurred on by this example and by the love of her late husband, a former steward of Bishop Alexander's household, Beatrice of Amundeville endowed an Austin hospital at Elsham in Lincolnshire. She had at least six sons, two of whom were also episcopal stewards and another who was diocesan treasurer and canon of the cathedral. Several of her sons confirmed or enlarged her grant to Elsham and one, Elias, gave alms to Saint Peter's, York, which was coming to be called Saint Leonard's after a church erected there by King Stephen. Elias also founded a leprosarium at Carlton. Coincident with these donations, another Lincolnshire canon, William of Saint Clare, the archdeacon of Northampton from 1133 to 1168 and a nephew of Bishop Alexander, founded the hospital of Saint John the Baptist and Saint John the Evangelist in Northampton. Finally, it is worth recalling that Bishop Alexander's uncle, Roger of Salisbury, was an active hospital benefactor and that Alexander's brother, Bishop Nigel of Ely, may also have founded hospitals. This intricate web of patronage was probably even more complex than this summary suggests.[35]

Beatrice and her family were successful, but not front rank, landowners. At little Aylesbury, in Buckinghamshire, four burghers of even more moderate means—Robert Ilhale, William atte Hide, William Fitz Ralph, and John Palnok—set up a local leper hospital dedicated to Saint John the Baptist. They donated a city tenement plus twenty-one acres of arable land and four acres of meadow, a handsome gift for four average men. Their example was unusually inspiring, for a very short time later a couple of other men in the same town together founded a second hospital and dedicated it to Saint Leonard. They gave fourteen acres for farming and two for pasture. This was quite an achievement for such a little place, but it may well have been the pattern throughout the country.[36]

Hospitals were expensive creations, although less so than monasteries. Basic funding was required for land, buildings, food, clothing, and staff. Undoubtedly some light agricultural and construction work was done by the patients themselves when they were not bed-ridden. The great hope, however, was that a host of small donations and bequests would supplement the original grants. In the early twelfth century this was a well-founded assumption, and, indeed, many minor gifts poured in. It was a good thing, too, for such contributions swelled endowments that would sustain hospitals through the leaner, less generous, years ahead. The church was exceptionally important, not only for the major contributions of its prominent leaders, but also for its persistent encouragement of lay donations. Archbishop Theobald, for example, began offering indulgences to generous donors, great and small. In later centuries this policy would have tragic consequences, but in Norman times it was a beneficial fund raising incentive.[37]

Turning from patronage to the daily routine is relatively easy because, whatever their affiliation, many hospitals patterned their internal organization on that of a religious community. Thus patients or residents, often clothed in a plain gray or russet tunics, were segregated according to sex. Required to follow a schedule that included periods of silence and devotions in chapel, the residents were under the direction of an administrative supervisor called a master or warden, who was often also a priest and counselor.

Adopting a religious model was not only the tradition of the times, it was also an eminently successful therapeutic device. Unlike today's patients, who are the passive recipients of professional solicitude, twelfth-century people actively participated in their own maintenance and recovery. They were expected to see themselves as vital members of a community, not as isolated individuals. Through prayer, patients were supposed to help each other and, indeed, to assist their relatives and friends and people everywhere. Many hospitals had definite local community responsibilities—educating and housing students, feeding paupers, maintaining bridges, and sponsoring commercial fairs. All this was both good theology and good psychology.

Consider, for example, the charitable work of Legarda, the widow of William of Apulia. After her husband's death this noblewoman and her attendants devoted themselves to the sick at the leper hospital of Saint Mary Magdalene, in Norwich. They worked among the patients and also begged in town for the hospital's financial support. One night in 1144, after the supposed martyrdom of a young boy in Norwich, Legarda saw a brilliant celestial display. She rushed to the hospital and arrived just as the residents were awakening for their midnight prayers. With great presence of mind she calmly led them outside to witness the starry phenomenon, a once-in-a-lifetime event. The point, however, is not the exceptional splendor of the sky in the silence of the evening, but rather that the sick folk were routinely keeping to their demanding rule and that able-bodied neighbors were regularly helping them.[38] Fortunately, newly discovered hospital regulations offer further insight into such daily routine.[39]

Since the responsibilities of hospital wardens were usually more administrative than medical, few early masters appear to have been physicians. One cannot be dogmatic about that, however. The elasticity of the term *master* is always confusing. When prefixed to a personal name it often indicated a physician. Moreover, after the Norman period several medically trained hospital masters can be identified.[40] Some wardens were monks appointed to manage their abbey's affiliated hospital, but other masters were even drawn from the ranks of hospital residents themselves. At Ilford, for example, the warden was required to be a leper.

Some hospital masters were talented, generous men, — but of little political importance beyond their own enclaves. Osmund, the hermit founder at Goathland, was one such self-effacing individual. Other administrators were of considerable national consequence because of the force of their personalities, the size of their institutions, or the scope of their family connections. For example, Robert, the master of Saint Peter's York from about 1121 to 1157, governed one of the largest and best endowed corporations of his day. He was one of those men who was both master of his own hospital and personally entitled to the designation of master by virtue of his prior training. The 200 patients in his care far outnumbered the religious controled by most abbots. Robert received directives from three different popes — Innocent II, Eugenius III, and Adrian IV — and was singularly vigorous in raising private donations for his hospital. He knew three kings of England and an exemplary roster of nobles and clergy. The endless stream of men and women who contributed to his institution reads like a *Who's Who of the North,* but also includes scores of lesser known, but equally generous, donors.[41]

The most interesting early administrator, however, was unquestionably Rahere, the founder of Saint Bartholomew's Hospital, near London.[42] He was a rather secretive, complicated man who came to prominence in King Henry's court. Tradition makes him a jester or minstrel, but no real evidence supports this. He was certainly a royal clerk and a canon of Saint Paul's Cathedral. His unusual name has a Flemish ring to it, but many of his connections seem to have been with Essex, where he may have been born and educated. It is tempting to think that Master Adelard of Waltham Holy Cross, or his son Peter, may have had some influence on Rahere's early training. One physician, the hermit Wulfric of Haselbury, was certainly an acquaintance. Like so many in that contradictory period, Rahere had pulled himself up from humble beginnings to modest prosperity, but in middle age he experienced a religious conversion, repudiated the blandishments of court life, and joined the growing company of royal bureaucrats who preferred to serve their creator rather than their king.

Rahere went off to Rome on pilgrimage, but, upon arrival, fell deathly sick and penitently vowed to build a hospital for the poor of London if he recovered. Shortly thereafter he had a vision, interestingly, on the Tiber island that supported the ruins of a temple to Aesculapius, the Roman god of medicine. The apostle Bartholomew appeared to him and gave detailed instructions for a new hospital at Smithfield, just outside London.

Rahere returned to England, sought help from King Henry and from the citizens of London, and in 1123 obtained a very large tract of land where he duly began his foundation. From that day to this Saint Bartholomew's has been one of England's finest hospitals. It was battered during the Reformation, but survived to flourish in the present when it is universally known as "Bart's." The strong columns and round arches of the romanesque priory church begun by Rahere still shelter worship services, and the founder himself rests on the elaborate, post-Norman, tomb in the nave. The church's continuous existence has happily preserved several exceptionally valuable records of the hospital's early activity.

Although Rahere probably began with the hospital, he actually established a joint foundation of a priory of Austin canons and a hospital for the poor. At the beginning he acted as canonical prior and hospital master. However, he soon saw the necessity of separating the two institutions. About 1133 a well-timed, valuable gift from Bishop Roger of Salisbury of the church of Saint Sepulchre, London, enabled Rahere to appoint a clerk named Hagno as independent warden of the hospital. From the wealthy living of Saint Sepulchre, Hagno was henceforth to pay fifty shillings a year towards the upkeep of the hospital.[43] By the time of Rahere's death in 1144 his hospital was well established, but the adjacent priory still had only thirteen canons. Perhaps this reflected the internal dissension that troubled the convent's second decade. The new prior, Thomas (1144–74), a former canon of Saint Osyth in Essex, made the unusual decision to appoint a layman as successor to Hagno, a businessman called Adam the Merchant (warden 1147–75/76).

The increasing separation of hospital and priory was an interesting development because it was contrary to the tendency in several other places, such as Saint Gregory Canterbury. Hospitals managed by Austin canons started out vigorously concerned with social work, but some gradually became absorbed in purely conventual matters. Over the decades hospitals such as Elsham, Hempton, and Angelsey so neglected their medical function that they became indistinguishable from normal Austin priories.

The site Rahere selected for Saint Bartholomew was unprepossessing, swampy land at the edge of a large cattle market. Criminals were executed nearby, and some of the new buildings were erected over a Roman cemetery. The spot had previously been pointed out to King Edward in one of his dreams, and the Confessor had prophesied that one day the area would be great before God, a suitably vague prediction that evidently came in handy some six decades later. An earlier chapel dedicated to the Holy Cross and used by the sick may have preceded Rahere's establishment and influenced his choice. His original hospital had a staff consisting of a master, eight brothers, and four sisters, and it was intended for the poor of the district. Interestingly, it also included a maternity ward, and special provision was made for the care of children whose mothers had died in childbirth.

Despite their involvement with Saint Giles-in-the-Fields, the citizens of London also generously responded to the needs of Saint Bartholomew. In particular a wealthy old Saxon named Alfune, who had already erected a church to Saint Giles in Cripplegate, teamed up with Rahere. He was a persistent, hard-working, no-nonsense man who had great rapport with many London merchants. Apparently he quickly took in hand the practical management of the hospital, especially with procurement of food, which was probably the single greatest expense. Alfune not only contributed his own money but each day approached traders to beg for additional food, alms, and materials for brewing beer. At one point he had an unpleasant encounter with a stingy butcher, and the historian of the house thought it was a miracle that the tradesman finally offered help. Geoffrey the Constable, a protegé of the viceroy, Roger of Salisbury, was, like his master, a generous benefactor, as were the members of the de Vere family of Essex and probably Countess Rose, the former tenant of the site.[44]

King Henry continued to encourage the hospital and the priory, giving them the valuable right of complete freedom from all taxes and obligations. Moreover, the king rather grandiloquently promised to defend the church "as if it were my own crown." His actual donations, cautious as always, seem limited to a few churches.[45] There was, however, some opposition to the hospital's activity and leadership, for Rahere increasingly took to confiding in servants and children rather than in local benefactors or fellow canons.

Some years after Rahere's death an anonymous writer at Saint Bartholomew decided to record the early days of the priory and the hospital. Some of his remarks are enigmatic, such as the reference to Raher's odd conversations and the report that he once noticed a valuable hymnal missing from the church and immediately rode to the Jewish section of London where he found it.[46] The writer was not concerned with recording surgical techniques or patient case histories, but he did depict the hospital as a large complex, well served by chaplains and nurses, and generous in providing daily meals of bread, beer, and cooked food. Most of all, the author sought to demonstrate that the saint himself, by performing miracles, was the best healer in the house.

Within this chosen format of recording miracles there is some very interesting information. For example, a carpenter from Dunwich in Suffolk named Adwyn had badly crippled hands and feet. He heard about the Smithfield miracles and resolved to go there. After arriving by ship he was carried directly from the Thames dockside to Saint Bartholomew's shrine and was then housed in its charity hospital. During his stay Adwyn was evidently expected to contribute something toward his own maintenance since he was partly supported by the alms of passersby. As time passed he regained a little strength and began to make simple artifacts, — such as distaffs for women, and loom weights. As his strength grew he turned to heavier tasks such as cutting wood. It has been suggested that he suffered from a classic case of chronic contractures caused by a fixed posture during prolonged illness. The condition healed gradually and was aided by a series of progressive occupational exericises. The priory annalist called the cure miraculous, but it seems more like an instance of successful physiotherapy. In gratitude Adwyn voluntarily performed carpentry for some London churches.[47]

The canon also describes how a well-known man from Norwich had once been bled but neglected to take care of himself afterwards. As a result he found he was unable to sleep. The problem offered the writer an opportunity to praise the measureless value of sleep. In poetic, almost Shakespearean, tones he mused that sleep "lightens the sweat of the day, refreshes a man for labor, and keeps whole and sound the nature of man and beast."[48] After enduring insomnia for seven years the Norwich man came to Smithfield and was healed. His experience highlights the skill the hospital staff must have developed in curing psychosomatic illnesses. The identification of poor hygiene after bloodletting as the cause of the distress is also interesting, for medieval doctors are often unfairly said to have treated only the symptoms of a disease, such as fever, rather than to search for its origin.

In another case Rahere personally ministered to the sick. He washed a woman's swollen tongue with water in which relics had been dipped. Normally his servant seems to have been charged with such tasks.

The average run of miracles is exemplified in the story of an unnamed paralytic woman. She was so shaken by palsy that she suffered the loss of her limbs. Though living beyond the Thames she was brought to Saint Bart's. After some time there, the power of the apostle healed her sickness, and she was able to return home, take a husband, and have children. The writer was very anxious to show that the hospital had a national reputation and attracted patients from all over the country. He was also interested enough in the former patients to follow their later progress, but it did not occur to him to describe the woman's course of treatment while at the hospital. The outcome seemed miraculous, and that was the major consideration.[49]

The treatment of leprosy presented special problems. A few scraps of medical technique can be gleaned from the excavations of a small hospital cemetery in Norwich. Skeletal remains from this period indicate that patients there had unusually low dental attrition, and it has been suggested that this resulted from their being fed moist foods which would not irritate sore mouths. It also seems likely that Norman practitioners had correctly observed that young children were particularly vulnerable to leprosy, for some institutions were established just for their care. Only within modern times had science rediscovered this childhood susceptibility.[50]

The affliction was rarely selective, however. People of all types were infected, even the richest and the most sheltered. Elder bishops, barons, and

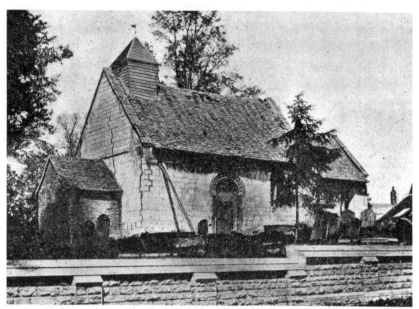

THE HOSPITAL OF SAINT MARY MAGDALENE, GLOUCESTER

Very early regulations for the daily routine of this lazaretto have recently come to light. This old photograph was made before 1861, when most of the nave of the hospital chapel was pulled down. The Norman doorway still survives, now incorporated in a truncated apse. By permission of the Bristol and Gloucestershire Archaeological Society.

monks were attacked as well as poor children. The disease was not well defined, however, and many types of skin lesions were tragically misdiagnosed as leprosy. Supposedly clinical analyses sometimes described it as highly contagious, venerally acquired, quickly developing, and even frequently congenital, for babies were born afflicted. Rather than specifying leprosy at all, these conditions seem to describe certain strains of syphilis. Such descriptions come from Salerno, but by at least the thirteenth century they were being repeated in England.[51] They represent another disastrous victory of theoretical study over careful observation. It certainly was not a mere academic question. Reliable estimates indicate that at the height of its virulence, which would be only about a generation after the end of our period, leprosy infected one out of every 200 Europeans.[52] Thus, its medical and social problems, in one form or another, would have been familiar to most people in Norman times.

Horrendous as the disease was, however, in early twelfth-century Britain it was not yet the great personal catastrophe it later became. The healthy

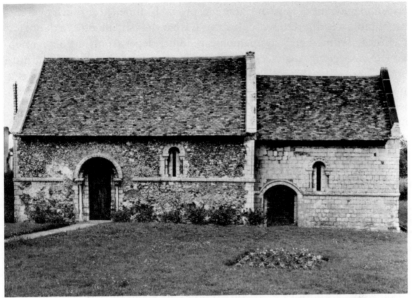

THE HOSPITAL OF SAINT MARY MAGDALENE, CAMBRIDGE

This picturesque chapel at Sturbridge, a mile from central Cambridge, dates from about 1150. Although the surrounding hospital buildings have disappeared and remain unexcavated, the small chapel is still periodically used for religious services. It accommodates a few dozen worshippers, perhaps an indication of the size of its vanished community. By permission of *The Cambridge Evening News*.

Anglo-Normans did not usually stigmatize or isolate their afflicted kin in the brutal, pointless fashion that characterized later peoples. Evidently, and rightly so, the condition was not then considered highly contagious. Lepers could be found living in their own homes with their own families or freely mingling with other people at markets, churches, and bridge crossings. Some lazarettos, like Saint Mary Magdalene at Sturbridge, a mile outside Cambridge, which still boasts an exquisite little Norman chapel, sponsored annual fairs which drew multitudes of visitors. The dubious liturgical practice of singing a Requiem for a stricken leper and then forever forbidding the victim the company of ablebodied people has not been found in early England, nor has the well-publicized requirement that lepers carry bells or clappers to warn of their approach.

It is true that lazar houses were placed outside town walls, but so were most hospitals. Lepers were certainly not popular figures even in the best of times, although pious souls like Queen Matilda somewhat ostentatiously saw them as affording opportunities to practice heroic charity. Inevitably lepers tended to gravitate toward one another, probably impelled as much by some sort of biblically directed sense that this is what they should do as a desire for uncritical, sympathetic companionship. Since leper's only income often came from begging, many less devout citizens considered them a public nuisance. Town officials probably found it convenient to deal with them as a concentrated group rather than as an endless series of individuals, and benefactors undoubtedly knew it was less expensive to donate properties outside of the towns. Some leper hospitals clearly welcomed people with other diseases and, when cured, they returned to the community. In fact, the leper hospital of Saint Mary Magdalene was built by Abbot Anscher of Reading Abbey (1130–35) "because of the large numbers of various infirmities among the poor at that time."[53]

Evidently, the public fear of lepers and the consequent ostracism of such unfortunates seem to be products of a slightly later age. Hospital regulations support this distinction. The early rule for the Dudston lepers did not castigate their condition, but rather, compassionately tried to insure their welfare. In fact, its exaggerted concern that they be submissive residents suggests a certain willful independence on the part of lepers. Again, the implication is that authorities were worried primarily about the lepers becoming a nuisance. Far different would be the precepts of later centuries. One rule echoed the harsh sentiments of the biblical Leviticus and began by reminding lepers that they had the most contemptible of all diseases.[54] It is no wonder that the thirteenth-century writer, Robert of Gloucester, wistfully thought that the days of Queen Matilda had been particularly good ones for lepers.

The silence of records makes it dangerous to generalize too readily, but the puzzling reality seems to be that lepers were better treated, or at least viewed less harshly, in Norman England than on the Continent or during later English history. Clearly, what people thought in one generation was not necessarily what their predecessors had believed. It is regrettable that datable evidence is so scarce, because it would be fascinating to uncover what brought about this terrible change in public and professional opinion.

Hospital masters like Rahere, Hagno, and Robert of York were the most visible members of hospital staffs and deserve special praise for helping to mold the favorable outlook of their times, but they were aided by many associates. At Saint Gregory's in Canterbury, for example, there were six priests and twelve clerks to serve the 100 residents at Saint John's and to teach the area schoolchildren. Moreover, all hospitals had numerous servants. Thirteen lepers enjoyed the services of three servants at Peterborough. In 1147 a wealthy leper named Robert de Torpel entered the hospital there and brought four of his own servants with him. He paid for his care by giving the monks two of his manors, on the condition that they maintain him and his servants and that he be buried as a monk. At this time Peterborough Abbey itself had sixty monks and about forty servants, some of whom were probably agricultural workers.[55]

Physicians were neither mentioned as members of hospital staffs, nor did they figure prominently in early hospital statutes. Most likely they were external consultants brought in as occasion required, rather than residents. York, however, had a disproportionately large number of physicians, probably because several of them worked directly for the great hospital. There are indications that nuns sometimes performed nursing duties, but usually their services are not recorded.[56]

Hospital regulations and donation charters pay more attention to creature comforts. Diets are outlined in some detail, although one cannot always be sure of the amounts. At Reading, for example, the daily ration included half a loaf of bread for each patient, but at Whitby it was a full loaf. Many early hosptials explicitly provided for one hot meal of meat or fish a day. Later establishments, such as Sherburn in Durham, founded in 1181, would cut down the full meals to three times a week and would emphasize eggs somewhat more. Everywhere special commemorations meant special meals. Sometimes donors gave alms for clothes or provided them outright. At Chichester, for example, the bishop gave the eight residents new woolen tunics at Christmas and new linen ones at Easter. Firewood was another frequent gift.

Most early buildings have perished, but a few others provide a glimpse of the standard groundplan. Although much of its fabric is later than 1150, Saint Cross Hospital, outside Winchester, still preserves the atmosphere of a wealthy medieval hospital where the residents are pensioners rather than chronically ill bed patients. A great courtyard is framed by the gateway, common hall, the large handsome chapel, and the wings of small attached apartments. Most hospitals had less impressive alignments and small frame clusters. Excavation reveals the extent of a few other structures. The leper hospital at Reading was built for twelve people and measured 110 feet by 50 feet, with the largest room 60 feet by 45 feet. The long hall at Saint John's Canterbury was 150 feet by 28 feet, and midway down its length a chapel sprang out at a right angle. Chapels were frequently attached to the dormitory for the sick in this way so that patients could participate in the solace of the Mass from their own beds. Thus there were few interior partitions and the groundplans often assumed a *T* or *L* shape. The *T* plan was favored by institutions catering to both sexes, for the post arm—the chapel—would divide the two groups.[57]

In 1154 hospital buildings thickly dotted the map of England and reflected the amazing transformation since 1066, or even since 1100. In sheer numbers alone hospitals represent a significant triumph of ingenuity over need. In immediate effect they reveal a whole new era in social welfare. At mid-century every person in England, whether lord, burgher, or serf, had a reasonable chance of obtaining both the professional services of a physician and the institutional shelter of a hospital. Few earlier or contemporary societies were so blessed.

It is tempting to award credit for this unique achievement to a single individual, and Henry I certainly presents the best case. The many hospitals that he and his family built or supported constitute the most notable segment of known facilities, but equally important was his persistent encouragement of other benefactors. Nevertheless, health patronage was a multitiered affair. Clergy and local leaders of all types began their own institutions quite independent of royal support. This widespread, intensely practical medical effort was the obverse of the coin of astrological science.

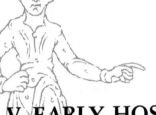

V. EARLY HOSPITAL
REGULATIONS

The daily practices of Anglo-Norman hospitals are almost as elusive as the personal crises of their vanished patients. Fortunately there are exceptions. The leper hospital of Saint Mary Magdalene in Dudston, just west of Gloucester, offers one opportunity to examine the daily routine of a medical facility. Its ancient rules have recently come to light, and they may well be the oldest known hospital statutes.

The succinct constitutions were boastfully attributed to the famous Bishop Ivo of Chartres (d. 1115). They were primarily intended to create good order and a purposeful life in a complex residential institution, rather than to outline medical requirements. Through the regulations Dudston fostered a monastic pattern in its community. Male and female patients followed regular schedules that included frequent prayer and periodic silence. Clothes were uniform, occasional fasting was prescribed, and members were forbidden to wander about unaccompanied. A formal promise of stability was required, and disciplinary measures were specified. The role of housemaster was so emphasized that the man became almost a father abbot to the patients.

On the other hand, the somewhat haphazard regulations do make ample allowance for physical infirmity. The bedridden were granted special privileges; sick travelers were entitled to a night's lodging; and everyone was allowed meat three times a week. The author was especially anxious that men and women did not become romantically involved with one another. Nevertheless, repeated injunctions against quarreling, and strikingly similar warnings from the hospital's benefactors, suggest that some of the thirteen residents may have been quite outspoken.

Dudstan's intriguing statutes have been preserved only because about 1350 a nameless, rather hasty scribe incorporated them into his large compendium of Llanthony Priory charters. In later years this two-volume work was called the *Registrum Magnum*. Together with many other valuable administrative books the cartulary eventually descended to Frances Scudamore, a troubled young woman who became insane shortly after her marriage to Charles Howard in 1771. When her husband, the duke of Norfolk, died in 1815, the duchess's interests required protection so her estate passed into Chancery receivership. The monastic records went to one of the masters for safekeeping and were never returned. It was just as well. Some less important documents released to her heirs were subsequently destroyed in enemy bombing during World War II.[1]

The best manuscripts are now maintained at the Public Record Office as part of the Chancery Masters Exhibits. Although there is considerable duplication among the eight Llanthony cartularies that were part of the Scudamore collection, the Dudston hospital regulations occur only on folio 75 of the first part of the *Registrum Magnum*.[2] Before examining their implications, the statutes should speak in translation.[3]

This is the rule of the sick of Dudston prepared by Ivo, the great bishop of Chartres, a man of the finest judgement.

1. Before all and above all obedience, patience, chastity, and common property must be observed by the sick.

2. The men should be separated from the women and not go into the house of the women, nor the women into that of the men without permission of the master.

3. On feast days a chapter should be held for the sick about noon time where faults can be corrected.

4. On Sundays, Tuesdays, and Thursdays let them eat meat, if possible. However, on other days they should abstain, unless the celebration of a feast supervenes.

5. However, if anyone should murmur about an insufficient supply of food or drink, let him be rebuked up to the third time. Afterwards, if he complains let his draught of beer be withheld from him until he makes satisfaction, because on account of complaining the sons of Israel died in the desert.

6. Even if the brothers and sisters possess more than two sets of clothing, let those also be of one color, namely black, white, or russet, not several different colors.

7. Those who are accepted as brothers and sisters should promise stability in the house and obedience to the master who presides.

8. The sick should not go outdoors alone, nor should they wander about the streets, but let them go with a servant or a companion in good order where they have been instructed to go.

9. The sick should not talk after compline, except for those who are altogether bedridden.

10. They should not talk in the church, except in the chapter when business affairs are being transacted.

11. If someone is denounced, prostrate let him seek pardon and humbly confess if he admits the complaint, or deny it if he was not guilty.

12. For the customary discipline of the master in such a case, let him impose a penance of beatings or fasting. However, if anyone refuses to accept discipline, as it is in the Cistercian Order, let him be expelled from the community.

13. If anyone falls into open fornication, let him be expelled from the community without any mercy.

14. If anyone is quarrelsome with the master, let him be sternly corrected; if he does this habitually, he should be thrown out.

15. Guests who are sick should be received charitably and entertained for one night according to the ability of the house.

16. At dawn everyone should rise for divine office and hear the matins of the day and of Saint Mary.

17. However, in place of matins laymen can say twenty-four Our Fathers. For each hour let them say the Our Father five times; instead of vespers, seven times; in place of compline, five times.

18. They should eat twice a day except on principal fasts, but at the proper time. All should know the Our Father, Hail Mary, and Apostles' Creed.

19. If anyone who is in good health should dedicate himself to the service of the sick, let him promise obedience and chastisty and live as the warden of sick directs.

20. No one should speak at table, unless about necessary things, nor should anyone presume to talk after compline except about necessary business of the house.

21. No one should go out into the town or village without the permission of the master and the master should carefully inquire into the business for which such a person goes.

22. And if anyone goes out before breakfast, he should come back for breakfast. And if he goes out after breakfast he should return for vespers. Whoever will not accept this regulation, should lose his special meal treat for twenty days.

23. No brother should be found with any sister, nor sister with any brother, in the cellar, or in the larder, or in the orchard, or in the field, under similar mealtime penalty of forty days.

Thus ends the rule of the sick prepared by Ivo, the great bishop of Chartres.

Dudston must have had many attractions in Norman times. The unusual, rather primitive, simplicity of its provisions bespeaks an open-minded atmosphere, as if the hospital were still experimenting with its direction. Unlike later statutes, its precepts are remarkable for their brevity, moderation, and tolerance. They contain no demeaning prologue castigating lepers for their disease; no declaration that suffering was God's will; no requirement that the inmates isolate themselves from society; and no demand that they pay for their own support. The commonsense Gloucester directives provide domestic arrangements, not health codes or moral strictures.

Dudston was a mixed community: male and female, young and old, rich and poor, lay and cleric, mobile and bedridden. Indeed, leprosaria were unique among charities in that they sheltered together people from all ranks of society. The poor had no monopoly on the disease. Distinctions, however, did not automatically disappear. Some patients were apparently better clothed than others and possessed more than the vestments traditionally distributed each Christmas and Easter. Priests also had greater prayer obligations than the laity.

The hospital groundplan and gardens can be fleetingly glimpsed in the precepts. There were separate quarters for the men and the women, but no special chapter room. Since they could hear each other talking, the bed patients and the ambulatory ones must have shared a common, single-sex dormitory. Moreover there were frequent chances to visit those seductive haunts of temptation—the cellar, the larder, the orchard, and the fields. Penalties for breaking household rules ranged from rebuke through enforced fasting to physical beating and possible expulsion.

Two problems particularly worried the author of the statutes: dissension in the house and illicit sexual relations. Even so, offenders were not severely punished unless their defiance became habitual. At first blush some provisions may seem unduly pessimistic, but that undoubtedly arises from the disciplinary style of this type of composition. Most rules sound harsh, but their real effect is determined by the grace with which they are enforced. Indeed, the moderator of any modern residential institution, be it a college, hospital, or hotel, knows that in every group, especially of long-term residents, some people are bound to be contentious.

The monastic derivation of these rules motivates the insistence on common prayer, ritual fasting, public confession, voluntary poverty, mealtime silence, guest hospitality, and member stability. Residents were not cloistered, however, and occasionally they had business in town. Nevertheless, the admonition that they move about the village in proper order suggests the paired strolling of novices so characteristic of all religious organizations. Yet some people were out alone and needed to rush back for breakfast or dinner. Townsfolk also came to the hospital. Apparently a fair number of nurses were expected, since they were specifically charged to obey the master and to be chaste.

Perhaps the strongest reflection of monastic principles appears in the exalted position of the warden, or rector, who was to be consulted about all affairs. However, the leper community also maintained something of the democracy of the monastic chapter because it, too, met in assembly, not only for the correction of personal faults, but also for group discussion of certain business decisions.

Dudston was a rather strict hospital, as such institutions went. Although it offers the clearest statutes, policies at other facilities were sometimes mentioned in charter donations and chronicle accounts. Thus, the food seems to have been better, or at least more plentiful, at Whitby whereas the clothing allowances were more generous, or more detailed, at Chichester. At Dudston the accommodations were in dormitories, but at Winchester each resident had a private room. Unlike Saint Cross, however, the color of one's clothing did not indicate specific status in the house. At Dudston each resident had the choice, provided it was consistent. Furthermore, patients there could sleep until dawn, as was common for most people, but at one of the Norwich hospitals the lepers had to rise for midnight office.

The most jarring note is the mandate not to quarrel about meals because a similar complaint brought death to the Jews in the desert. However, all administrators know that food is the main cause of institutional complaint in any age. Fortunately, the ever increasing holydays must have steadily, and expensively, improved the daily menu. Above all, the sick were urged to be obedient and patient. This was useful, if uninteresting, advice. It sums up the low-key approach of the author, who was thinking of residence in the leper hospital as a lifelong commitment.

The actual history of Saint Mary Magdalene Hospital is intimately tied to the experience of Llanthony Priory, upon which it was dependent, and to the generosity of the earls of Hereford, who were among its earliest patrons. The relationship to Bishop Ivo is not as straightforward, especially since the precise foundation date of the center is so clouded. However, the hospital is considerably older than scholars once thought.[4]

Llanthony Priory had quite a complicated history of its own. In 1103 William, a knight-turned-hermit, was joined in the wild mountains of Monmouthshire by Ersinus, a former chaplain to Queen Matilda. Within five years they built a church dedicated to Saint John the Baptist, adopted an Augustinian rule for their followers, and received several endowments from Hugh de Lacy, an important local baron. At intervals Austin canons joined them from Aldgate, Colchester, and Merton priories. King Henry, Queen Matilda, and Bishop Roger of Salisbury all supported the remote foundation, which soon included more than forty religious. An especially learned man, Robert de Bethune, became second prior sometime before 1129.

Following the king's death the burgeoning house suffered from Welsh attack, and in 1136 many canons took refuge at Hereford where Prior Robert had reluctantly become bishop in 1131. Their exile was supposed to be temporary, but Miles of Gloucester, a powerful royal official and regional magnate, gave them land near Gloucester for new buildings and the bishop added other endowments. By 1137 the community was installed in what came to be called Llanthony Secunda. Although Miles, earl of Hereford from 1141 until his death in 1143, despoiled the priory during the troubled days of Stephen's Anarchy, his descendants later rectified his depredations. A handful of canons had remained in Monmouthshire, however, and the two priories continued in uneasy affiliation until 1205. Many years later, in 1481, in a full turnabout, Llanthony Prima became dependent upon the Gloucester establishment.

Earl Miles's father, Walter, the constable of Gloucester, probably founded the Dudston hospital and linked it to Llanthony. He had been a trusted minister of William Rufus and Henry I from 1097 until his retirement to Llanthony and death there in 1128. Some time earlier he had given Llanthony half of the manor of Great Barrington, Gloucester. This endowment and its use for the Dudston poor were confirmed by his son Miles before 1135 and by his grandson Earl Roger in 1151x1155. Roger also added modest grants of his own: food, clothing, and firewood for thirteen lepers, and a house and land for a resident chaplain. He concluded his charter with the strong warning that if any of the residents became contentious and incorrigible the offender was to be expelled from the community and replaced by another person. This caution was remarkably similar to one expressed in the Dudston rule itself.[5]

It is not surprising that patrons regularly backed the administrative staff in quarrels with hospital residents, but the internal divisions at Dudston reappeared in yet a third context. An undated reconciliation between the master and the lepers specifies quite precisely the rights of the chaplain and his clerk. Evidently the intention was to insure that the general funds of the residents were not diminished, but the priest came off quite well in the agreement.[6]

By at least 1155 the sick (*infirmi*) at Dudston were recipients of an annual royal gift of twenty shillings.[7] The stipend does not seem to have originated with Henry II, but it was not recorded in the lone earlier pipe roll of 1130, either. Presumably it began sometime thereafter. The first known doctor at the hospital seems to have arrived by 1160.[8]

Since the statutes at Dudston were attributed to Ivo of Chartres, it would seem axiomatic that the hospital must have been founded before his death in 1115. Although it has been demonstrated that the institution did exist before 1128, the prior chronology is not so simple. Bishop Ivo was one of the truly great men of his era—a poet, preacher, and politician, an Austin canon like the clerks at Llanthony, a friend of kings and common people. Only the charm of his personality rivaled the depth of his wisdom. He was most acclaimed for studies in canon law, especially for a decretal collection called the *Panormia*. In fact, the bishop was so famous that lesser writers often appropriated the authority of his name for their own compositions. Thus it is possible that the identification of these statutes with the bishop was merely a literary fiction.

Three alternatives present themselves: (1) Ivo composed this code for Dudston; (2) Ivo composed the code and, sometime later, Dudston adopted it; (3) Ivo's name was attached to a code he did not originate. That final connection could have been made as late as 1350, but would be more likely in the generation after 1115 when Ivo's fame was at it height.

The new British hospitals of the early twelfth century were usually completely autonomous institutions or separate facilities tied to monastic establishments. Except for Saint Peter's York, which did create daughter hospitals, they rarely had any formal connections with any other medical centers. Fundamental policy was normally determined by a nearby sponsoring house, often an Austin priory, or by a dominant lay patron. As might be expected, many hospitals therefore gradually modeled their own internal regulations on those of traditional religious communities. This was particularly true of leprosaria, which inevitably catered to permanent residents. Quite pragmatically, hospital founders often worried more about building and endowing their creations than providing them with detailed statutes.

Nevertheless, drafting constitutions was a major intellectual preoccupation of the period, and it was bound to have ripple effects. There were several reinterpretations of the ancient rule of Saint Benedict, including that of the new Cistercian order, and many other rules were devised in accordance with the vague and newly popular principles of Saint Augustine. Those hospitals that did draw up statutes naturally stressed basic ideas like common property, uniform dress, scheduled prayer, and strict obedience to a master. Within this shared heritage the details varied a great deal from place to place. The spread of one constitution to several facilities, however, was quite untypical.

Although differing hospital codes eventually became quite commonplace, up to now the earliest known examples have been the rule drawn up by Raymond of Puy, Grand Master of the Hospitaller Knights from 1125 to 1153, for their enormous general-purpose hospital of Saint John of Jerusalem, and the rule drawn up by Bishop Raymond of Montpellier (1129–58) for the leper hospital of Saint Lazarus, Montpellier.[9] These longer constitutions bear little resemblance to the terse guidelines for Dudston. Abbot Anscher of Reading (1130–35) also provided special, hitherto unrecognized, instructions for the leper hospital attached to his abbey. He was quite detailed in listing the patients' dietary and clothing allowances.[10]

Interestingly, regulations also exist for a second Gloucester leprosarium, Saint Margaret and Saint Sepulchre. This was founded about 1150, perhaps by the monks of Gloucester. Its rule, now partially illegible, was drawn up by an abbot of Gloucester in Anglo-Norman French, not Latin, and seems to date from about 1200. Despite proximity to Saint Mary Magdalene of Dudston, this institution also had quite different precepts that primarily concerned prayer and dietary specifications.[11]

Ivo of Chartres had had extensive experience with several phases of organizational planning and hospital design. Before becoming bishop in 1090 he had been prior of the new Austin monastery of Saint Quentin of Beauvais and had prepared a set of customs for that house. Its substance was understandably quite different from the Dudston code.[12] Later, perhaps working with Count Theobald III, he established a great shelter for lepers, Le Grand Beaulieu de Chartres. In 1110 he wrote to Countess Adela of Blois, a sister of Henry I of England, and mentioned the prior of his hospital, a man named Helias. The context suggests the prior had been in office for some time.[13] In succeeding years many lords increased the hospital's endowment, including King Henry, who gave a large subsidy of ten pounds a year and remitted tolls for its commerce within his realm.[14]

Evidently Bishop Ivo personally prepared a set of statutes for this hospital, but unfortunately its text has disappeared. Although the regulations were not explicitly mentioned in any Chartres record or in the bishop's own voluminous correspondence, by 1208 the constitution at Le Grand Beaulieu was already considered ancient. This document, probably Ivo's composition, was replaced in 1264 by a reforming bishop of Chartres, who set down new, rather lengthy statutes. They have little in common with the Dudston provisions.[15]

Ivo's original ideas attracted more favorable attention in Normandy, at the leper hospital of Saint Giles of Pont Audemer. A facility was established there about 1129x1135 by another Beaulieu supporter, Waleran, who was the count of Meulan from 1118 to 1166. However, it may have succeeded an earlier lazar house built on the same spot by his father, Robert. King Stephen credited his predecessor with a major share in the creation of the second hospital, and Henry's chief justiciar, Roger of Salisbury, was an important benefactor. Waleran's foundation charter stated quite definitely that Saint Giles was to follow the rule (*religionis regulam*) drawn up by Bishop Ivo of Chartres. Surely this was the Beaulieu constitution. Saint Giles was not subordinate to the Chartres hospital, but the two did cooperate, and Master Gerald of Beaulieu was present at Pont-Audemer in 1135 when Waleran put his gifts on the altar.[16]

It thus seems unlikely that Ivo prepared totally different rules for hospitals at Chartres and at Dudston. More probably he, or indeed some later intermediary, sent a version of the Chartres statutes to Dudston in the same way that an edition was used at Pont Audemer.

King Henry's own role in the exchange is shadowy, but nonetheless important. He confirmed Walter's gift to Llanthony, heavily endowed Beaulieu, and was actively involved with Pont Audemer. Clearly leprosy, the so-called royal disease, was never far from his thoughts. It is not inconceivable that he encouraged a Chartres-Dudston-Pont Audemer connection.

Bishop Ivo was quite familiar with conditions in England. Besides his valuable friendship with the king, he also knew Anselm of Canterbury from as far back as their student days at Bec. Moreover, he corresponded with other British leaders, including Queen Matilda. His books were quickly copied in monasteries and cathedrals throughout the country and used by chroniclers like William of Malmesbury. A large contingent of English students even trained at his cathedral.[17] However, no other information ties him to Dudston.

Of all the later candidates who might have transmitted Ivo's ideas, Robert de Bethune seems the most likely. The youngest son of a knightly family, Robert was first educated by his older brother. Robert became a local schoolmaster, but later went to Laon for further study. Eventually he experienced a religious conversion and retired to Llanthony. He was soon prior, and then bishop, of Hereford. Robert was a cosmopolitan, well-traveled man who had frequent, if mixed, dealings with the Gloucester dynasty of Walter, Miles, and Roger. He had an outstanding reputation for learning and sanctity, but no modern biographer has yet analyzed his career or cataloged his acts. He did, however, regularly aid Llanthony and confirm donations to Dudston.[18]

There are indications in the Dudston rules that their author, whoever it was, thought of more than one hospital when drawing them up. At one point the rules state that visitors should be entertained "according to the ability of the house" and, at another, patients are forbidden to go into the "town or village" without permission. Both phrases suggest a multipurpose generality.

Furthermore, there is the curious statement, "If anyone refuses to accept discipline, as it is in the Cistercian Order, let him be expelled from the community." The anomaly is the reference to the Cistercian Order. Ivo was a great exponent of Austin values, but he is not known to have been intimate with the new reformers at Cîteaux. That abbey was founded in 1098, but its unique organizational plan and important daily customs were only worked out some years later by the Englishman Stephen Harding. The dating of these decrees is very complicated, but the first references to them apparently come as late as 1114x1119. The Dudston entry would therefore seem an interpolation in Ivo's possible text. If not, it is one of the earliest references to the Cistercians' own constitutions.[19]

Moreover, the Cistercian White Monks established their first English houses at Waverly in 1128 and Rievaulx in 1131, long after Ivo's death. It is difficult to see how the small Dudston community could have been expected to be familiar with Cistercian practice—which included possible punishment with a cord whip, or "discipline"—before any house of the order was even erected in Britain. William of Malmesbury, however, was conversant with Cistercian reforms before 1125 and discussed Stephen Harding, who was from Sherborne in Dorset, in his *History of the Kings of England*.

Until more of the questions are resolved, it seems reasonable to conclude that the present text was not specifically composed by Ivo for Dudston.[20] However, the brevity of its precepts and their freedom from condescending restrictions argue for an early date. This supports Ivo's claimed authorship, but suggests a slightly later transmission of the statutes to Gloucester. The Llanthony cartulary may thereby enshrine not only regulations used at Dudston, perhaps quite soon after its foundation, but also the substance of the original Beaulieu precepts. In any event, they do offer considerable insight into the residential side of a typical Anglo-Norman hospital.

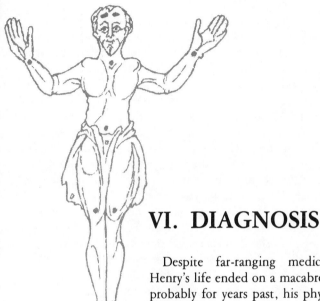

VI. DIAGNOSIS

Despite far-ranging medical interests, King Henry's life ended on a macabre note. In 1135, and probably for years past, his physicians were desperately trying to bring his weight under control. In late November he foolishly disregarded their dietary advice, feasted on a meal of lampreys, and died, as contemporaries said, from the resulting ill humors. He expired on December 1, 1135, at Lyons-la-Foret in Normandy, in his sixty-seventh year. Perhaps doctors had expected the worst. The portents had been very bad. Wulfric of Haselbury had predicted that Henry would never return to England alive and the famous eclipse of 1133, which so many scientists had recorded, occurred at midday on August 2 while the king was asleep aboard ship crossing the Channel.

In death the mighty lord did not rest well, either. Despite the removal of his intestines, brains, and eyes for separate burial at Rouen and the salting of the rest of his body for transport to entombment at Reading Abbey, his corpse still fouled the air. Henry of Huntingdon, who recorded all the details with morbid relish, would even have readers believe that an attendant, called in to sever the king's head and extract his brain, died of the stench and thus became "the last of the great multitude that King Henry slew."[1] Even then, the royal remains relentlessly continued to decompose in the weeks before they could be returned to England. Finally, centuries later, at the dissolution of the monasteries, Henry's bones were further desecrated, and now his tomb is unidentifiable. The only merit the early chronicler could discover in the monarch's wretched decay was that it was yet another graphic lesson urging all mortals to be contemptuous of the mutability of beauty, fortune, fame, and power, and to fix their eyes on the eternal glory of God alone.

Perhaps some further reflections can now be added. Realization that the passing of princes could also be horrible was cold comfort to their poorer subjects, but it did remind people of their essential equality before the great mysteries of life. Miracles, marvels, and medicine also cut across the distinctions which artifically divided people. Kings might reign and rule, but real depth in the social order came from the responsible daily contacts of relatively obscure individuals. Henrican physicians, like their friendly associates the scribes, teachers, and chaplains, may have been bit players in the outstanding contests of the age, but their very existence then gave added stability and essential service to society. Now their gradual rediscovery illumines yet one more strand of the astonishingly complex web of human relations that once held the Anglo-Norman world together.

The unprecedented multiplication of physicians, manuscripts, patrons, and hospitals demonstrates that some long-dormant seeds of medical practice were finally putting forth shoots. A pervasive emphasis on realistic observation and rational casuality fed these awakening interests. Even the cutting of the king's body would have produced some anatomical knowledge.

In life Henry's positive support for health care frequently surfaced. His wives' charities, his own possible thaumaturgic beliefs, his pleasure in stimulating company, his insatiable curiosity, his need to placate restless subjects, his late desire for penance, the horrifying growth of leprosy, and the unpredictable visitation of famine and disease — all these things focused his attention on medical matters. The subject was probably a low-priority item for him, but it was a real one nonetheless, and Henry's actions were immediately beneficial.

One should not exaggerate twelfth-century knowledge, skill, or concern, however. Much of that era's practice was ignorant, brutal, and downright silly. Much was also extraordinarily generous. On the other hand, eight hundred years later, in our own world of escalating medical costs, impersonal service, physicians' slowdowns, and the yet uncured common cold, we should not be unduly critical. The post-Conquest era, after all, may still have something to tell us about geriatric care — the outstanding Anglo-Norman success and our glaring scandal. Then too, modern medicine, which sometimes merely substitutes placebos for incantations, may be rapidly reverting from curative to custodial care with its proliferation of nursing homes, retirement villages, and drug rehabilitation centers.

One unsettling question remains. Was the medical achievement of Henry's reign a uniquely "golden moment" in social progress or did it have enduring effects? Certainly much of the bloom faded in Stephen's time.

Nothing indicates that kindly but devious, weak-willed monarch ever had any special interest in health care. No physician can be linked with him, and no hospital claims him as founder. The extent of the so-called anarchy of his reign is a matter of endless historiographical debate, but clearly many prominent and many faceless officials quickly left government service after his treacherous disgrace of Roger of Salisbury. The civil war between Stephen and the Empress Matilda was quite real, and its death and destruction canceled many projects.[2]

Fortunately, the broad-based hospital construction program survived the plague of war. Medical education, scientific research, and popular attitudes were more adversely affected. Naturally there were other factors at work—such as the triumph of theoretical studies, the hardening of class divisions, and the moderating of religious fervor—but war was the terrible catalyst that made life uncertain for everyone. In medicine this callousness would appear in the conversion of hospitals to convents and in the increasing persecution of lepers.

The final lesson is not defeat and decay, however, but rebirth and renewal. Henry and his followers had done too much for all their work to be lost. Above all, they had set a standard and an example for succeeding generations. A snowy-white caladrius looked upon English health care and decided that it should eventually thrive, after all.

APPENDIX I

A Directory of Anglo-Norman Physicians, 1100–1154

This whole study originated in the gradual realization that an unexpectedly large number of men had practiced medicine in early twelfth-century England. Accordingly, each time I chanced upon the trace of such a healer I dropped his reference into a special file. Eventually I systematically searched surviving records to uncover as many physicians as possible. Excavating these shards of past lives, and seeing obscure individuals slowly reappear from oblivion, proved rewarding.

This appendix lists each physician, that is, each medicus, who can be found by name in England before 1154. Initially, I counted only the practitioners of King Henry's era, but later this seemed unduly restrictive, especially as I grew curious about the health care actually available within a single lifetime—a span closer to sixty years and a period nicely covered by the combined reigns of Henry I and Stephen. Although it may be somewhat awkward to enroll one practitioner who is only vaguely detectable sometime between 1148 and 1166 and yet to exclude another who is precisely traceable to a year such as 1157, this decision does maintain the realistic and significant interval 1100 to 1154.

My investigations soon led to the extraordinary compendium of Charles H. Talbot and Eugene A. Hammond, *The Medical Practitioners in Medieval England: A Biographical Register* (London, Wellcome Historical Medical Library, 1965). Their scholarship has been invaluable, and I salute their prodigious research. However, new documents and better editions of old sources have become available since they first blazed the trail. I have been able to extend their efforts quite substantially, identifying thirty-nine new healers, revising accounts of twenty-five others, and deleting ten superfluous entries. The current tabulation stands at eight physicians for the Saxon centuries, eleven for the years 1066–1100, and ninety for the epoch 1100–54.

As Talbot and Hammond observed, there is precious little that can be said about each man, and even those scraps usually involve tenurial or fiscal arrangements rather than medical activities. Nevertheless, in their corporate strength and personal idiosyncrasies, these Anglo-Norman physicians still reaffirm the unusual concern for health care which characterized their society.

1. MASTER ADAM, YORKSHIRE

Master Adam is mentioned as a charter witness four times in mid-century Yorkshire. Although his appearances are difficult to date, the first is interesting because Adam attested a grant of William, son of Henry of Beningbrough, to the poor men of the hospital of Saint Peter's, York. With the doctor were Robert, his "fellow"—evidently another medicus—and Elias, his nephew.[1]

The second charter, Walter Engelram's gift of a large pasture to Rievaulx Abbey, can be dated 1158x1167.[2] The two other transactions, gifts of Richard Fitz Roger and Roger Fitz William to Guisboro Priory, cannot be pinpointed.[3]

About 1180 Master Adam Medicus was signatory to two charters granting Durham Priory part of the church of Bilborough in Lincolnshire, but this was probably a different physician.[4]

[1] *Calendar of Charter Rolls*, pp. 444–45. Talbot and Hammond, (p. 1), suggest a date 1100x 1150, but the deed can only be placed 1143x1177. The first witnesses are Robert, dean of Saint Peter's, and Robert, master of the schools. There were two deans Robert, 1143–57 and 1157–86; the schoolmaster drowned in 1177.
[2] *Rievaulx Cartulary*, p. 51. For the date see pp. 260–62. *E. Y. C.*, (2:60, no. 713), published this with the date 1160x1170.
[3] *Guisboro Cartulary*, 1:232–33. Talbot and Hammond suggest a date of about 1180 and think that the above grant and these two were associated with a second Adam medicus.
[4] Talbot and Hammond, p. 1 (entered as a third Adam medicus).

2. MASTER ADELARD

Master Adelard (Athelhard, Ailred) was a very distinguished secular canon attached to the collegiate church of the Holy Cross in Waltham, Essex. According to a late twelfth-century legend, Earl Harold Godwinson had become partially paralyzed in 1060, but his own personal physicians and others "brought by entreaty or payment from all parts of the country" were unable to assist him. Somehow the German emperor learned of Harold's distress and sent Adelard, a famous Flemish educator and physician, to heal him. Finding that his own medical arts were also unsuccessful, Adelard, "unlike lying and deceitful doctors," advised the earl to pray to a holy relic kept at Waltham, a sacred crucifix found in Somerset some years before. In a short time a cure supposedly resulted. In gratitude Harold greatly enriched the church of the Holy Cross and added ten new canons, including Adelard, to the Essex house.[1]

The physician was a native of Liège and had studied at Utrecht, the center of a considerable intellectual revival in the mid-eleventh century.[2] He helped Harold prepare statutes and customs for Waltham and became master of students there. After Harold's victory at Stamford Bridge, the king prayed at Waltham on his way to Hastings, but this time the famed cross supposedly turned away from him. Some accounts say that after the battle his body was returned to Waltham for burial. The church then passed to the control of the bishop of Durham, but it was despoiled by the Normans, especially William Rufus, who carried many of its treasures back to Normandy. Master Adelard evidently made a detailed inventory of these depredations.[3]

He may also have written a commentary on Quintilian. A thirteenth-century catalog of the monastery's library lists such a work by a Master Adelard.[4] The catalog also reports a collection of medical books, mediocre but for a few duplications of Herbert of Durham's holdings. Adelard had at least one son, Master Peter, but there is no certain indication that he also became a physician, although he did follow his father's religious and scholarly interests by becoming director of the Waltham school (by at least 1124).[5]

Adelard lived well into the twelfth century, and his death on October 5 was commemorated in the liturgical calendar at Durham.[6] Scribbled at the end of another Durham manuscript was a short mortuary roll requesting prayers for three Waltham canons: Dean Walter, Master Adelard, and Osgoto.[7] Since Walter was still active about 1108, the deaths probably occurred sometime thereafter.

[1]Birch, *Vita Haroldi*, pp. 117–19. Not in Talbot and Hammond.
[2]Stubbs, *Waltham Abbey*, p. x.
[3]Ibid., p. 32.
[4]James, "Essex Monastic Libraries," pp. 41–44.
[5]The name Peter medicus appears in Bedford, Canterbury, and Leicester in this period; the Canterbury doctor had a son, John medicus.
[6]Stubbs, *Waltham Abbey*, p. xxi.
[7]B.L., Ms. Harley 491 (an early twelfth-century collection of historians), fo. 47v. For Dean Walter, see *V.C.H., Essex*, 2:166; *Regesta*, 2, no. 1984; *Aldgate Cartulary*, p. 224. The next dean, Geoffrey, appears by 1113x1116; *Regesta*, 2, no. 1109. The other canon may be Osgood Cnoppe, who, with Ailric, the schoolmaster, supposedly brought King Harold's body back from Hastings. Evidently several men taught at Waltham simultaneously.

3. AILRED OF RIEVAULX, YORKSHIRE

Ailred was born in 1110, the descendant of a distinguished Saxon clerical family from Northumbria. He was educated at the Scottish royal court, but later became an Austin canon at Kirkham. At age twenty-four he transferred to the new Cistercian community at Rievaulx. He was chosen first abbot of Revesby, serving from 1143 to 1147, and then elected abbot of Rievaulx. Ailred wrote many historical and devotional books and regularly served the sick. He was frequently unwell himself, suffering intensely from arthritis and stones, to ease whose passage he took many baths each day. Ailred's biography was written recorded by a brother monk, faithful disciple, and fellow physician, Walter Daniel, who recorded instances of the abbot's treatments and his use of such simplistic practices as putting two fingers into a man's mouth to induce vomiting. Ailred was renowned throughout the country for his sanctity, and he sometimes preached at great occasions, such as the canonization celebration for Edward the Confessor. He died on January 12, 1167. He was never formally elevated to sainthood, but the Cistercians kept his cult and feast day. He is easily the most famous man on this roster of physicians, with the possible exception of Pedro Alfonso. Although he was called a medicus and regularly worked in the infirmary, the title may have been intended as a compliment rather than as a mark of professional training.[1]

[1]The literature on Ailred is quite extensive, and his writings are steadily appearing in translation. The most interesting account of his life is by his friend Walter Daniel, *The Life of Ailred of Rievaulx*. There is a modern biography by Ailred Squire, *Ailred of Rievaulx*. (London, 1976). Talbot and Hammond include neither Ailred nor Walter Daniel in their register.

4. ANDREW, KENT

Andrew is mentioned early in 1108 as part of the retinue of Bishop Gundulf of Rochester when that prelate appointed the first abbess of Malling.[1] Gundulf was then in his eighties and quite sick in that the last year of his life. Andrew, perhaps a monk of Rochester, was obviously a physician in attendance on the ailing prelate. At some earlier time Gundulf had been unsuccessfully treated by an unnamed doctor for eye trouble.

[1]Sawyer, ed., *Textus Roffensis*, 2, fo. 198r. Not in Talbot and Hammond.

5. ARNOLD, SUFFOLK

Sometime between 1153 and 1164 Peter Boterel gave the monks of St. Melanie of Rennes a peasant named Godwin, the reeve of Nettlestead in Suffolk.[1] Most of the village attested the grant, including Arnold medicus and Andrew, "the son of Arnold." Since Arnold's name appeared between those of two priests, he was presumably a cleric himself. In order to attest, his son would probably have been at least twenty, so Arnold would most likely have been practicing as early as 1133x1144.

[1]B.L., Additional Charter 28331. This has been published several times: *Historical Manuscripts Commission, Seventh Report*, p. 579; Lowndes, "A History of Hatfield Regis," pp. 121–22 (abstract); Douglas, *Medieval East Anglia*, p. 232, no. 17; Douglas and Greenaway, eds. *English Historical Documents.*, pp. 844–45. Not in Talbot and Hammond.

6. BALDWIN, ESSEX

Baldwin medicus attested two charters of Richard of Beauchamp, an adherent of Earl Gilbert of Clare (1138–48), giving land to Colne Priory, a dependency of Abingdon Abbey in Essex.[1] He witnessed after the chaplains and clerks and was probably a layman. Baldwin may have had a son, William, who appears 1176x1183.

[1]*Colne Cartulary*, pp. 30–31, nos. 58, 59; for William, son of Baldwin, see no. 61, Picot, Gloucester. Not in Talbot and Hammond.

7. BERNARD, DURHAM AND YORK

Mention of Bernard medicus is made three times in Durham and York about mid-century: with Bishop William of Saint Barbara attesting for the nuns at Newcastle (about 1144);[1] with Dean Robert of York attesting for Hexham (1143x1153);[2] and with Ernald de Percy attesting for Guisboro Priory (1142x1154).[3]

[1]Offler, ed. *Durham Episcopal Charters*, p. 132; incorrectly recorded by Dugdale, *Monasticon*, 4:488.
[2]*E.Y.C.*, 1:349, no. 450.
[3]*Guisboro Cartulary*, 1:232; *E.Y.C.*, 1:91, no. 746, incorrectly dated 1154x1165 since one of the witnesses was Augustin, prior of Newburgh (1142–54). Talbot and Hammond, p. 25.

8. BERTRAM, LONDON

Bertram medicus was on a long list of witnesses to an undatable gift of Simon Fitz John to Saint Paul's Cathedral, London.[1] Most of the signatories who are known elsewhere fall in the 1132–54 period. Bertram had a low ranking in the list and may have been a layman.

[1]*Historical Manuscripts Commission, Ninth Report*, p. 68; Talbot and Hammond, p. 26.

9. CLAREMBALD

Royal physician, priest, canon at Exeter and London, 1108/17–30; see Chapter 3.

10. EDWARD, DEVON

Between 1161 and 1170 Roger de Nonant gave Saint Mary of Totnes land called Stretcheford, formerly held by his teacher, Master William Buzon, who flourished about 1137. Before William, the land had been held for a long time by the physician's sons, Edward and Geslinus, and earlier still by the physician himself. Edward must therefore have practiced about 1140, or earlier.[1]

[1]Watkin, *History of Totnes*, 1:55; Talbot and Hammond, p. 40, without date.

11. MASTER ERNULF, ELY

Master Ernulf medicus was a physician associated with Bishop Nigel of Ely. Sometime during that prelate's episcopate (1133–69) "Master Ernulf and John the doctors" attested one of his charters for the priory at Ely Cathedral.[1] The unusual wording suggests that the scribe, and perhaps the physician himself, may have deliberately wished to highlight Ernulf's more advanced professional training. About 1140x1145 Ern[ulf], or Ernald, medicus pledged ten marks to the building of the cathedral.[2] It was a generous contribution, but only one-quarter the size of some other gifts. Since it is unlikely that a monk would possess such capital, Ernulf must have been a secular clerk or a layman. In fact, the monks at Ely had a long history of employing laymen as their medical officers.[3]

Without referring to his medical skill, but simply signing himself Master Ernulf, he also attested a 1135x1158 confirmation of Bishop Nigel.[4] The similarity of fellow witnesses to the fund contributors identifies this master with the physician. In view of the imaginative spelling used during this period, it should also be noted that a Master Arnald twice attested with John the Physician in 1162x1169.[5] Ernulf's professional career may thus have stretched from 1133 to 1169; at least it covered the years 1145 to 1162.

[1]Miller, *Abbey and Bishopric of Ely*, p. 285.
[2]*Liber Eliensis*, p. 335.
[3]*V.C.H., Cambridge*, 2:205.
[4]Gray, *Priory of Saint Radegund*, p. 75. Nigel's charter confirmed a grant of William Le Moyne of 1135x1136, which was also confirmed by King Stephen. Gray suggested a date of 1157x1160 for Nigel's charter, but earlier dates seem more likely. Certainly the grant was made before 1158, the last appearance of William, the archdeacon.
[5]*Liber Eliensis*, pp. 381–83. Not in Talbot and Hammond.

12. ERNULF, LONDON

Ernulf medicus attested a charter (1140x1144) of Geoffrey de Mandeville, earl of Essex, for Holy Trinity Priory.[1] Iwod medicus witnessed with him. Geoffrey may have been in his last illness when this deed was issued.

[1]This writ has been printed several times: Round, *Commune of London*, p. 101; *Aldgate Cartulary*, p. 190; Douglas and Greenaway, eds., *English Historical Documents*, 2:953. Talbot and Hammond, pp. 43–44.

13. FARITIUS

Cellarer at Malmesbury Abbey in 1078; abbot of Abingdon 1100–17; important royal physician; see Chapter 3.

14. GEOFFREY, BERKSHIRE

In 1108 Geoffrey medicus attested a charter of Robert, count of Meulan, for Abingdon Abbey. One of several physicians associated with the Beaumont family, Geoffrey was also one of several doctors known to have had dealings with Abingdon Abbey in the time of Abbot Faritius.[1]

[1]*Abingdon Chronicle*, 2:102–3. Not in Talbot and Hammond.

15. GEOFFREY, NORFOLK

Geoffrey medicus witnessed two grants for Castle Acre Priory in Norfolk about mid-century.[1] His dates are very difficult to establish, but some of his fellow signatories are known before 1160.[2] Since "Geoffrey the master of Saint Julian's Hospital" occurs in the same cartulary, this raises the possibility that the doctor was also the hospital administrator.

[1]B.L., Ms. Harley 2110 (cartulary of Castle Acre Priory), fos. 10d, 11d. Talbot and Hammond, p. 422, noted the second text only.
[2]Carthew, *The Hundred of Launditch*, 1:128.

16. GERVASE, DURHAM

The name Gervase medicus appears both before and after its owner's death. At some point, King David of Scotland (1123–53) had granted him lands that later passed to the nuns of Saint Bartholomew, Newcastle.[1] Before 1158 William de Granville, baron of Ellingham, endowed the bridge across the Tyne with certain lands on the condition that Gervase the Physician and his heirs become tenants. Again the date of the gift is uncertain, but the bridge existed before 1137. This land was still in the family in 1220x1230 and was then held by the physician's grandson, Gervase, son of Ranulf.[2] Before 1158 Gervase medicus also attested one charter for Durham Priory involving the same William de Granville and, between 1156 and 1174, another for Roger de Merlay.[3]

A possible, but hapless, allusion to Gervase's practice may be detected in the fate of Emma de Granville, William's wife. The villagers of Embleton, where she lived, knew her well and passed along her story. Emma became afflicted with a grievous but unspecified malady and suffered a kind of feverish ague, boiling one moment and freezing the next. She lost a great deal of weight and scandalized some people by removing her clothing when the fever seized her. Unfortunately, the zeal of un-named medical attendants aggravated her condition, and she became a complete cripple, leaning on two crutches. Finally, the lady resolved to make a pilgrimage to the spot where Saint Cuthbert had died. After approaching as near to his cloistered church as a woman was allowed to go, she was miraculously cured with the help of the hermit Bartholomew of Farne (d. 1193).[4]

Like other physicians, Gervase may have been an author and bibliophile. Before 1163 a second list of Durham library books was made. The section on medicine con-tained the entry "Liber Gervasii medicii."[5] Whether this meant a book was given by Gervase or was written by him is uncertain. Alternatively, an entirely different indivi-dual could have been involved.

There are, in fact, further references to men called Gervase. In the mid-twelfth century an eloquent clerk of Durham named Master Gervase revisited Paris where he had once studied. He became ill there, but could not be healed by any of the city's famous doctors. He then returned to Durham and was soon healed by the local her-mit, Godric of Finchale. Evidently this Gervase later went to Guisboro Priory. In a separate incident, Lawrence, the prior of Durham, addressed a letter to someone named Gervase. Perhaps one, or both, of these men can be identified with the physician.[6]

In any event, between 1154 and 1174 Bishop Hugh gave some of the land of Ger-vase medicus to Durham Cathedral, presumably after the physician's death.[7] In 1166 the lands granted to Gervase by King David reverted to the English crown; the most likely reason for this would be the doctor's death. Oddly enough, the royal exchequer continued to account for these lands under Gervase's name from 1166 to 1178, and again in 1201.[8]

[1]Hardy, ed., *Rotuli Chartarum*, p. 87a, citing an entry from 1201 that records this gift.
[2]Oliver, ed., *Newcastle-Upon-Tyne*, pp. 67–68.
[3]Greenwell, ed., *Feodarium*, p. 104; Hodgson, *Northumberland*, 2:142.
[4]Craster, "The Miracles of Farne," p. 99, and "Miracles of St. Cuthbert"; Reginald of Durham, *Cuthbert*, ch. 62; Bateson, *History of Northumberland*, p. 13.
[5]Botfield, ed., *Catalogues of Durham Cathedral*, pp. iv, 6. Talbot and Hammond (p. 56) rather freely phrased this as "at his death he bequeathed all his medical books to Durham priory."
[6]Reginald of Durham, *Godric*, pp. 62, 452.
[7]*Brinkburn Cartulary*, p. 180.
[8]Hodgson, *Northumberland*, 3:3, 9, 10, 12, 14, 15, 18, 20, 21, 28, 301.

17. GILBERT, LONDON

Between 1128 and 1138 William, the dean of Saint Paul's Cathedral, London, gave John the Physician and his heirs the land that Wilfrid the canon had once given the cathedral in Aldermandbury. Last in the long list of witnesses to this deed is Gilbert medicus.[1]

[1]*Historical Manuscripts Commission, Ninth Report*, p. 676; Gibbs, ed., *Charters of St. Paul's*, pp. 172–73. Wilfrid was evidently still holding the land in 1128; Davis, "London Lands," pp. 49, 57. Talbot and Hammond, p. 56.

18. MASTER GILBERT, PETERBOROUGH

Before 1130 Master Gilbert medicus of Peterborough (Burgh) witnessed a charter of William Olifard and Hugh Olifard for Thorney Abbey.[1] Hugh Olifard had succeeded to his father's responsibilities by 1130.[2]

[1]Cambridge University, Additional Ms. 3020 (a cartulary of Thorney Abbey), f. 79. Not in Talbot and Hammond.
[2]*Regesta*, 2, no. 1685a; *31 Henry I*, pp. 50, 48, 85.

19. GILBERT OF FALAISE, NOTTINGHAM

In the Pipe Roll of 1130, under the section for Derby and Nottingham, Gilbert of Falaise, medicus, accounted for forty-five silver marks for the lands and daughter of John of Monte Caluino. He paid the treasury four pounds and still owed twenty-six more.[1] Gilbert was clearly a layman — and a fairly rich one — to be able to pay such a high relief for his wife and lands. Apparently they had no children, for his sister was his heir. She married Manasser Bisset, the steward of Henry Plantagenet.[2]

[1]*31 Henry I*, p. 8. Not in Talbot and Hammond.
[2]Lewis C. Loyd, *Origins of Some Anglo-Norman Families*, Harleian Society 103(1951):15.

20. GREGORY, MALMESBURY

Ernulf de Hesdin, a powerful lord in Normandy and Oxfordshire, suffered a serious disease of the hands. He consulted Gregory, the famous physician of Malmesbury Abbey, but the monk could not help him. Abbot Godfrey (1091–1106) then located some balsam in the tomb of Saint Aldhelm, rubbed it on the knight's hands and cured him.[1] Ernulf suffered other difficulties, however. He was accused of treason in 1095 and lost most of his land, but he later proved his innocence and then went on crusade and died at Antioch.[2] His death date helps to establish that the monastic doctor Gregory flourished at the turn of the century.

[1]William of Malmesbury, *G.P.*, pp. 437–38. Talbot and Hammond, p. 66–67.
[2]Lennard, *Rural England*, p. 69; Douglas, *The Norman Fate* (Berkeley and Los Angeles: University of California Press, 1976), p. 171. Ernulf would seem to have died in 1099, but perhaps he made a later trip to the Holy Land, for his wife Emmelina may have been working at his request as late as 1100; *Regesta*, 2, p. 406, no. 438a (1086x1100).

21. GREGORY, WARWICK

Henry of Beaumont, earl of Warwick (d. 1119), confirmed a gift to the collegiate church of Saint Mary of Warwick, and a long list of associates attested his grant. Included were Theulf, bishop of Worcester (1115–23), Gregory, medicus of the earl, and Ralf, the teacher of Henry's son.[1] Although there were merely sixty houses within its walls, Warwick was a thriving place. It had an ancient school, a priory of the canons of the Holy Sepulchre, erected at the request of pilgrims returning from Jerusalem, and a nearby leper hospital established before the end of Henry I's reign. Gregory was evidently the personal physician of the earl.[2]

[1]P.R.O., Ms. E 164/22, fo. 8 (Warwick College Cartulary); printed in Dugdale, *Monasticon*, 6:1326, with a slightly different witness list. Not in Talbot and Hammond.
[2]*V.C.H., Warwick*, 2:97; for revised datings see *M.R.H.*, p. 401.

22. GREGORY, STAFFORDSHIRE

Ralph Basset of Drayton (d. 1166) confirmed some gifts to Canwell Priory in Staffordshire, founded about 1142. Among the witnesses were Hugh, the archdeacon of Leicester (c. 1147–58) and Robert, the son of Gregory the Physician. Robert's father would have been active about twenty or more years earlier, 1127x1138.[1]

[1]Dugdale, *Monasticon*, 4:107; *V.C.H., Staffordshire*, 3:213–14. Conceivably, Gregory could easily have centered his activities in Drayton, in Cambridgeshire, rather than Staffordshire. Not in Talbot and Hammond.

23. GRIMBALD

Layman; important royal physician 1101–38; see Chapter 3.

24. MASTER GUY, MERTON

Master Guy was a renowned Italian educator who became an Austin canon of Merton Priory at its foundation in 1114. While there, he was ordained a priest and achieved a reputation for great skill in hearing confessions, consoling penitents, and helping sufferers. In one instance the prior himself experienced relief from his distress as Guy prayed for him and treated him *unde velut peritus medicus*. About 1120 Guy was made first prior of Merton's daughter-house at Taunton, but he failed as an administrator. He was a zealous, almost fanatical person who indulged in prolonged fasting and self-punishment. Guy was extremely generous to the poor, but in a disorganized way that offended many potential supporters. He was reportedly quite happy to be recalled to Merton thereby relieved of his responsibilities, but in 1123 he was sent to Cornwall to establish a new house at Bodmin. He died there following spring. A short time later a canon at Merton composed a biographical sketch about the priest. The author clearly considered his subject a saintly man who was even able to calm storms by his prayers. The canon was not very interested in Guy's early life or medical background, but he did stress his hero's special success as a counselor.[1]

[1]Rainald of Merton; for the date of Guy's death see Brett, *English Church*, p. 9. Not in Talbot and Hammond.

25. HALDANE, LINCOLNSHIRE

Haldane medicus is known only through his son David, a priest of Toynton, in Lincolnshire, who received a grant from William de Roumare.[1] David held land in fee from William as early as 1166.[2] Since he was an ordained priest, David must have been born at least twenty-four years earlier, and his father must have flourished about 1142. David later gave part of the land to the Templars and in 1200 part was confirmed to his daughter Isolde by King John. Haldane's name indicates Scandinavian ancestry. It appears several times in area records, but one cannot be certain that these references are to a physician.

[1]B.L., Harley Charter 55 E 14; published by Stenton, ed., *Danelaw*, p. 357. Talbot and Hammond (p. 422) oddly identify the holding as Fottingdon, Norfolk.
[2]Farrer, *Honors and Knights' Fees*, 2:161.

26. HENRY, YORKSHIRE

Henry medicus, a physician of Yorkshire, is mentioned four times in the mid-twelfth century. Talbot and Hammond suggest he may have been in the service of Henry de Lacy, which is certainly possible. His name appears twice in Henry's company, but also twice with Jordan Foliot and twice with Alice de Quentin.[1]

[1]Henry witnessed in connection with the following deeds: once for Kirkstall Abbey (c. 1150x1159), *E.Y.C.*, 3:192–93 (for some unknown reason Talbot and Hammond [p. 71] dated this 1154x1159); twice for Nuns Appleton (c. 1163), *E.Y.C.*, 1:422–24 and (1147x1153 or 1163x1170) *E.Y.C.*, 1:425, also in Dugdale, *Monasticon*, 5:653; and once for Pontefract (1159x1170, or 1137x1158, depending upon whether one signatory, Osbert, the archdeacon, was still a church official rather than the layman he later became), *E.Y.C.*, 3:214–15, also in Dugdale, *Monasticon*, 5:126. Talbot and Hammond say Henry witnessed another grant to Pontefract and cite *E.Y.C.*, 3:193, but I cannot find it there.

27. MASTER HENRY OF BOLWICK, NORFOLK

This Henry was in Norfolk at the very end of the period. In 1153x1168 he attested as "Henry the medicus of Bolwick."[1] Much later, 1175x1195, he attested as "Master Henry de Bolwick"[2] and at four other times simply as "Henry of Bolwick."[3]

[1]Stenton, "St. Benet"; J. R. West, *St. Benet of Holme, 1020–1210, Norfolk Record Society Publications* 2(1932):94.
[2]Carthew, *The Hundred of Launditch*, 1:75.
[3]West, *St. Benet*, p. 96 (1153x1168), 98 (1153x1168), 115 (1175x1186), 174 (1190x1203). Henry of Bolwick is not listed in Talbot and Hammond.

28. MASTER HERBERT, DURHAM

Before 1153 Master Herbert medicus donated twenty-six different books, mostly medical studies, to the monks of Durham Cathedral Priory. Several of these tracts still exist, and all the titles demonstrate his up-to-date scientific reading.[1] Unfortunately, nothing else about Herbert has yet been discovered for the years before 1153. There are some additional related details, however. Sometime between 1153 and 1195 a "Master H. medico" attested a grant of a chaplain of Bishop Hugh of Durham.[2] At an undetermined point in the century, a "Master Herbert medicus" attested a charter of Alexander Fitz Ralph of Brankeston for Durham.[3] Then, in 1196, an Alan of Aanetorp indicated that his toft in Beverley, Yorkshire, had previously belonged to a "Herbert medicus."[4] Talbot and Hammond thought this Herbert was a local leech in the village of Beverley.[5] However, Beverley was more substantial than they seem to suggest, and it was also an enclave of Durham's jurisdiction. In 1130 and 1150 King David associated with a "Master Herbert Scotto."[6]

[1]See Chapter 2 for a discussion of this large gift.
[2]*Guisboro Cartulary*, 2:303, no. 1128. This could also be Hugh medicus.
[3]Hodgson, *Northumberland*, pt. 3, 2:148; Raine, *North Durham*, p. 140. One of the other witnesses flourished about 1199.
[4]*Feet of Fines, 7 Richard I (1196)*, p. 137.
[5]Talbot and Hammond, p. 88.
[6]Lawrie, ed., *Early Scottish Charters*, pp. 75, 184, 209, 210, 121, 214. For some other Master Herberts, see Raine, *North Durham*, p. 26 (1146), p. 82 (1156), p. 83 (1173).

29. HUGH, ABBOT OF CHERTSEY

Hugh medicus was a monk of Saint Swithun's, Winchester, before being elected abbot of Chertsey. He evidently confined his interests almost exclusively to his own monastery, and there is no record that he ever even attested a royal writ. In 1116 he did join an ill-fated expedition to Rome, accompanying Archbishop Ralph of Canterbury, Bishop Herbert Losinga of Norwich, and William Corbeil, who was then only a canon of Saint Gregory's Hospital, Canterbury. Before they left France, Archbishop Ralph took sick, developed a facial ulcer, and almost died. After crossing the Alps Bishop Herbert became ill and had to be left at Piacenza. The others fared as poorly: there were earthquakes in January, the Po flooded, Rome was in revolt under an antipope, and the weary travelers never did see the true pope. Chroniclers report that the noted physician Hugh tried hard but was unable to help his patients, perhaps because they were being justly punished for their sins of pride and for intended bribery of the curia. The "punishments" continued. At Dover, in 1118, William Corbeil took sick and had nightmares of devils tormenting him. In 1119, at Rouen, Archbishop Ralph suffered a stroke and remained partially paralyzed and unable to speak properly for the last three years of his ife. Bishop Herbert eventually returned to Norwich, but died there in 1119. Abbot Hugh's later encounters were left unchronicled.[1]

[1]Hugh the Chanter, *Church of York*, p. 50; Eadmer, *H.N.*, p. 239; Bethell, "William of Corbeil," pp. 145–59. Talbot and Hammond, p. 90.

30. MASTER HUGH, KENILWORTH

Master Hugh medicus and his nephew Warin were among the witnesses to a deed made by Richard, the son of William Barton. The document confirmed a grant that Richard's uncle William de Furneaux had made of the church of Barton Seagrave, Northamptonshire, to Kenilworth Priory.[1] The original gift was made earlier than 1125, when it was included in a general royal confirmation of Kenilworth's possessions.[2] Robert de Furneaux, another uncle whom Richard prayed for, was still alive in 1130.[3]

[1]B.L., Harley Ms. 3650 (Kenilworth cartulary), fo. 25. Talbot and Hammond, p. 422, for no apparent reason, date this to the reign of Henry II, but this seems rather late. A fellow witness with Master Hugh was Savarinus, possibly the Savarinus who was later (1134–47) prior of Horsham, in Norfolk. Land at Barton Seagrave was later held by the physician, Master Ralph de Beaumont.
[2]*Regesta*, 2, no. 1428 (c. 1125); *Regesta*, 3, no. 418 (1136x1139).
[3]*31 Henry I*, p. 27

31. HU[GH], ESSEX

Maurice of Windsor, the steward of Bury St. Edmund's and his wife Edith (d. 1141x1156) made a grant to the nunnery of Wix in Essex, founded 1123x1133. The deed was attested by a "Hu— — medicus."[1]

[1]Dodwell, "Charters Relating to the Honour of Bacton," p. 162. Brooke, in "Episcopal Charters for Wix Priory," (pp. 47–50) contends that the charter is a forgery, but Dodwell claims it reproduces the "substance and detail of earlier deeds." Not in Talbot and Hammond.

32. HUGH, TOTNES

The small town of Totnes in Devon attracted a remarkable number of doctors. Edward has already been listed, but two others, Hugh and John, were also neighbors and contemporaries. Hugh seems to have appeared first. Roger de Nonant, Richard Balzan, and William Galenis attested separately with the two practitioners, but in the charter Hugh witnessed, William called himself a knight.[1] When he appeared with John, he described himself as a monk. There were two Roger de Nonants (1088–1130) and (1134–70), so it is difficult to distinguish between them. William de Nonant appeared in the first charter and Roger's wife Adeliza and his son Guy in the second. Both these men attested royal writs as early as 1102x1105, and Guy was still active in 1121x1135.[2] Doctor Hugh therefore would seem to have flourished about 1130.

[1]Watkin, *History of Totnes*, 1:36, 42. Not in Talbot and Hammond.
[2]*Regesta*, 2, nos. 735a, 1391, 1958. Adeliza may have been Roger's second wife, as a wife Matilda appears with him in 1102x1105.

33. HUGH, LEWES

Guy de Menchecurt confirmed a deed involving the priory of Lewes and Walter of Ditchling sometime around 1140. Hugh medicus attested as one witness and Master Leo as another.[1]

[1]*Lewes Cartulary*, 2:63; Guy is known to have attested a charter of John de Chesney (d. 1146), ibid., 2:47. Master Leo was known at Lewes in 1110; ibid., 1:155. The cartulary editor suggested a date of about 1150 for Guy's charter, but it could have been much earlier, since Leo attested. Talbot and Hammond, p. 90.

34. HUGH, YORKSHIRE

Hugh medicus attested a grant of Dean Robert and the chapter of York Cathedral for Rievaulx Abbey between 1142 and 1155.[1] Then in 1154x1181 a "Master H. medicus" attested another charter with many York officials.[2] Among the books belonging to Rievaulx in the twelfth century was a book of medicine that had once belonged to Hugh of Beverley, perhaps the same man as the physician.[3]

[1]*Rievaulx Cartulary*, p. 170; Talbot and Hammond, p. 90. *E.Y.C.* 9:215, no. 129, dated this 1163x1169, but one of the signatories, Hamo, the vice cantor, became full cantor in 1155.
[2]*Guisboro Cartulary*, 2:303; not in Talbot and Hammond. This may have been Master Herbert.
[3]James, *Manuscripts in Jesus College*, p. 48; not in Talbot and Hammond.

35. HUGH, NORFOLK

Hug[h] medicus attested a charter of Ralph de Friville for Castle Acre Priory, Norfolk, about mid-century. Another witness was Walter of the hospital, perhaps a master, or less likely, Walter medicus from Norfolk.[1]

[1]B.L., Ms. Harley 2110 (Castle Acre cartulary), fo. 55. Not in Talbot and Hammond.

36. HUMPHREY, HERTFORDSHIRE

Humphrey medicus attested a 1153x1185 grant of Hertfordshire lands to the Templars by Thomas of Buckland.[1]

[1]Lees, Records of the Templars, p. 219. Not in Talbot and Hammond.

37. IWOD, LONDON

Iwod medicus attested a charter of Geoffrey de Mandeville, earl of Essex, for Holy Trinity Priory, London, about 1140x1144. With him attested Ernulf medicus; this may have been during Geoffrey's last illness.[1]

[1]See note under no. 12, Ernulf, London. Talbot and Hammond, p. 95.

38. JOCELIN, CHICESTER

Jocelin medicus attested a writ of Bishop Hilary of Chichester (1147–69).[1] A Master Jocelin gave medical books to Cirencester Cathedral, but this may have been Bishop Hilary's nephew, who was commonly addressed as Master Jocelin.

[1]Chicester Cartulary, p. 68, dated it 1147x1163 and Mayr-Harting, Acts of the Bishops of Chichester, p. 95, dated it 1154x1163.

39. JOHN

Bishop of Bath 1088–1122; see Chapter 3.

40. JOHN, LONDON

Between 1128 and 1138 William, the dean of Saint Paul's, London, gave John the Physician and his heirs the lands that Wilfrid the canon had given the cathedral in Aldermandbury. The last witness to the deed was Gilbert medicus.[1]

[1]See note under no. 17 Gilbert, London. Talbot and Hammond, p. 101.

41. JOHN, TOTNES

John was one of three doctors in Totnes of whom there is mention in the early twelfth century. Edward and Hugh were his professional colleagues. John, who appears a little later than Hugh, perhaps about 1135, attested a deathbed grant of the knight, William de Lingeure, to Totnes Priory.[1]

[1]Watkin, History of Totnes, 1:42. Talbot and Hammond (p. 100) date the charter merely to the twelfth century. Unfortunately, the Lingeure family kept the name William in successive gener-

ations, so this particular instance cannot be distinguished. However, four of the other witnesses to this transaction also signed a grant of about 1130, the one attested by Hugh, the physician. Thus John and Hugh were almost exact contemporaries.

42. JOHN, ELY

John was associated with Bishop Nigel of Ely. During his episcopate (1133–69) "Master Ernulf and John the doctors" attested one of his charters for Ely.[1] Evidently some distinction was being made between the training or status of Master Ernulf and the lesser achievement of John, a simple medicus. Between 1139 and 1160, and twice between 1162 and 1169, John attested other charters of Nigel. The last two were also witnessed by Master Arnald (Earnald), possibly Ernulf medicus.[1]

[1]Miller, *Abbey and Bishopric of Ely*, p. 285. Not in Talbot and Hammond.
[2]*Liber Eliensis*, pp. 382–83.

43. JOHN, ESSEX

John, a medicus of Essex, received a penny a day from the royal exchequer from at least 1156, the date of the earliest pipe roll, until August, 1171. In 1168–69 and 1169–70 the rate was halved for some reason, but it climbed back again in 1170–71 and remained stationary until John's presumed death on the feast of Saint Lawrence. His penny payment was then awarded to a Master Edward for the remainder of the year. In 1171–72 Edward's yearly total jumped from 30 shillings 5 pence to 40 shillings 10 pence. Evidently the new man could increase his benefits in a way the old retainer never did.

In 1156–57 John was called *minutor*, in 1157–58 and 1158–59 *medicus*, in 1159–60 and 1160–61 *Dubbedent*, and from 1161 to 1171 *Adubedent*. The first word means "bleeder," the second "physician", and the third and fourth perhaps mean "dentist." A penny a day was a standard rate for many wages and charities.[1]

[1]For the yearly payments of 30 shillings 5 pence see the pipe rolls of Henry II, beginning *3 Henry II*, p. 72, and then 4:132, 5:3, 6:10, 7:63, 64, 8:68, 9:21, 10:36, 11:15, 12:122, 13:151, 14:151, 15:122, 16:103, 17:118; for Edward, 17:118, 18:39, 19:11. The daily rate was first noticed by that genius of records, John Horace Round, in "The Earliest Essex Medical Man," pp. 337–38. The title of his article, but not its substance, is now outdated by the discovery of Baldwin and Master Adelard as medici in Essex. Not in Talbot and Hammond.

44. MASTER JOHN, OXFORDSHIRE

John medicus attested three mid-century deeds concerning the property of Eynsham Abbey, but in only one did he use the title master.[1] He is a rather late figure who gains admission into this directory only by the skin of his teeth.

[1]*Eynsham Cartulary*, 1:81, no. 85 (1163x1180); 83, no. 88 (1150x1195, the time of Abbot Godfrey, as master medicus); 105, no. 126 (1150x1195); Dugdale, *Monasticon*, 3:22. Not in Talbot and Hammond. The cartulary editor gives vague, estimated dates, e.g., c. 1180.

45. JOHN, YORKSHIRE

John medicus of York attested a charter of Eustace de Merc (1150x1170) for the obscure convent of nuns at Covenham, Lincolnshire.[1]

[1]*E.Y.C.*, 1:426; Talbot Hammond, p. 101. A doctor named John later attested a number of deeds for Guisboro Priory, but he was probably a different individual; *Guisboro Cartulary*, 1:27, 225, 226, 238, 2:v, 17, 105, 120, 197 (datable to 1230), 235–37.

46. LAMBERT, YORKSHIRE

For at least three decades Lambert was associated with the Lacy family of Yorkshire. Shortly after 1135 he first appears in records as "Lambert the medicus of Clithero" attesting a deed of Ilbert de Lacy, an important baron, who had just been restored to the honor of Pontefract.[1] Clithero, in Lancashire, was usually considered part of the Pontefract fee. It had a great Norman castle by 1102 but was the site of a major Scots victory in 1138. After Ilbert's death in 1141, Lambert became part of the retinue of Henry, the baron's brother. By 1145 the physician had witnessed one of Baron Henry's writs along with Bishop Ralph of Orkney and the bishop's son, Paulinus, an important cleric who was later to be master of the greatest hospital in York.[2] Thereafter, Lambert's traces become easier to follow. He was signatory to Henry de Lacy's charter endowing the new Cistercian abbey of Kirkstall, founded in 1147, and he attested four other transactions between 1143 and 1155.[3] In one late attestation he emphasized his clerical as well as his medical status, and in another he called himself a physician of York.[4] Five more of his attestations are also known.[5] All told, he witnessed fourteen grants with members of the Lacy family.

[1]Farrer, *Lancashire Pipe Rolls*, pp. 388–89 (1135x1141). Talbot and Hammond, p. 200.
[2]*E.Y.C.* 3:229, no. 1547. The editors dated this 1144x1160, but Bishop Ralph, who was consecrated in 1109, is not otherwise known to have attested after 1144.
[3]*Kirkstall Cartulary*, p. 50 (1147x1153); *E.Y.C.*, 3, no. 1544 (1145x1155); *E.Y.C.*, 12:103–5, nos. 74, 75, 76, (all datable 1143x1154).
[4]*E.Y.C.*, 3, no. 1772 (1160x1177), no. 1531 (1160x1170).
[5]*E.Y.C.*, 3, no. 1491 (1141x1177), no. 1506 (1155x1177), no. 1567 (1165x 1175, this could also be 1155x1177), no. 1673 (1154x1177), no. 1773 (1160x1177). A Lambert medicus appears in Yorkshire in 1190–1210, *E.Y.C.*, 1:228, no. 295, but this is probably another physician.

47. LUCIAN, ESSEX

Lucian the Physician attested the marriage settlement that William de Yspania, an Essex knight of Henry I, made for his bride, Lucy.[1] Among the early medical books at Saint Albans's Abbey was a *Tractatus Luciani de Febribus et de Epidimale morbo*. Since no other medical writer named Lucian is known at this time, this might well be Lucian of Essex.[2]

[1]B.L., Additional Charter 28347, dated in the catalog as at the time of Henry I and Stephen; printed, *Historical Manuscripts Commission, Seventh Report* (1878), p. 579; W. S. W. and A. W. [sic], "Exampled of Medieval Seals," *The Archaeological Journal* 13(1856):62–64; Powell, "Essex Fees of the Honor of Richmond," facsimile and text; the charter has a well-preserved seal attached. William of Spain was known as early as Henry's reign, but as late as 1196x1198 he, or a man of the same name, is mentioned with Robert Fitz Mengi, another individual involved in the bridal dower. By then William had a new wife, Agnes; *Clerkenwell Cartulary*, nos. 68, 69, 70, 71, 204. Talbot and Hammond, p. 205, merely listed Lucian as a twelfth-century doctor. For William in Henry's time see *E.Y.C.*, 5:230.
[2]Hunt, "Library of St. Albans," pp. 25–77. Hunt thinks this charter is probably 1153x1172, but that seems late to me.

48. MARK

Mark medicus was present when Archdeacon John of Bayeux (elected bishop of Sees in 1124) gave Bernard, the king's scribe, the land and houses Gisulf had once held in London. Bernard and several other witnesses were court clerks, so Mark may also have been a member of the royal entourage.[1]

[1]Round, "Bernard the King's Scribe," p. 428; Heales, *Records of Merton Priory* p. 10; *Regesta*, 2, no. 1364. Talbot and Hammond, p. 210.

49. MELBETHE, CUMBERLAND

Before 1126 Waltheof, the son of Gospatric, earl of Dunbar, gave land at Allerdale in Cumberland to his physician, Melbethe. The descendants of this practitioner later took the name de Bromfield from one of the villages included in the gift. Waltheof, evidently the same lord, entered Crowland Abbey in Lincolnshire and was abbot there from 1126 to 1138. Melbethe was probably a layman, since he was specifically excluded from the advowson of Bromfield.[1] It is likely that he had a son, Ralph, who can be found about 1150.[2]

[1]Dugdale, *Monasticon*, 5:585, Prescott, ed., *Register of Whetherel*, p. 384; Nicholson and Burn, *History and Antiquities*, 2:165. For Abbot Waltheof see *H.R.H.*, p. 42. Talbot and Hammond, p. 215.
[2]Grainger and Collingwood, eds. *Register of Holm Cultram*, p.29.

50. MILES, NORTHAMPTON

Miles medicus was an innocent witness at a complicated family estate settlement. At some point between 1136 and 1141 Roger de Chesney (d. 1141) gave a mill at Dallington, Northamptonshire, to Evesham Abbey with the consent of Eva, the wife of Walter de Chesney. Their lord, Simon, earl of Northampton (1136–53) confirmed this grant. Miles appears in an undated charter of Walter of Chesney and his wife mentioning the same mill.[1] After 1154 Eva and Walter made another gift to Evesham, which was attested by, among others, "John of Wales" and his brother, Miles.[2] Since a "John medicus" later appears with Ralph, another member of the large Chesney family, it is tempting to think that this particular Miles was also the physician, making this a case of brother practitioners.[3]

[1]*Evesham Cartulary*, 1:79, no. 80 (in which the editor suggests a date of 1141x1148); Dugdale, *Monasticon*, 3:22. Talbot and Hammond, p. 216, merely place Miles in the mid-twelfth century.
[2]Dugdale, *Monasticon*, 3:24.
[3]Ibid., p. 22.

51. NIGEL

Nigel medicus was an important landowner who was recorded in Domesday Book as holding estates directly of the king in nine different counties. Although it is likely that he served the Conqueror and that these properties rewarded good service, no precise connection can be made between him and King William. Many of the lands Nigel held in 1086 had once belonged to a wealthy priest named Spirites, but there is no reason to think that the physician was himself a priest. Certainly he was far from generous to the church. His only gift seems to have been to the Norman abbey of Saint Mary of Monteburgh, to which he gave a five-hide estate in Somerset worth 100 shillings. Nigel held nine manors in Hereford and one in Worcestershire from Saint Guthlac's Priory but seems to have been an uncooperative tenant. He also held the wealthy church of the royal manor of Calne in Wiltshire and was prebendary of the royal college of Dover, which passed to Canterbury in 1130. In Wiltshire his lands totaled forty-three hides and three virgates and were worth 35 pounds in 1086, a handsome sum. Other smaller holdings were in Kent, Hampshire, Gloucestershire, Devon, and Shropshire. Evidently Nigel was still active in 1107x1128.[1]

Among the many estates credited to Nigel medicus in 1086 were four hides of the manor of Wistanstow, Shropshire. In King Edward's time these had been held by Spirites the priest. There was also a prebendal church in Wistanstow, which the Confessor had given to a certain Godric Wiffensune. This man continued to hold the same prebend under the Conqueror and under Earl Roger of Shrewsbury (1071–94). After Godric died the earl gave the church to his own physician, a clerk named Nigel. When this Nigel died, Earl Hugh (1094–98) the son of Earl Roger, bestowed the living on the canons of the college of Saint Alkmund in Shrewsbury. It passed from them about 1145 to the new Austin priory of Lilleshall. In the thirteenth century these events were recorded in the abbey cartulary, and the Wistanstow practitioner was specifically identified as the earl's doctor.[2]

At first glance it is tempting to identify Domesday Nigel with Nigel of Wistanstow. One medieval reader of the cartulary certainly did so, for a different hand from that of the main scribe noted in the top margin the Domesday information that Nigel medicus held four hides from the king in Winstanstow. However, not all details of the two lives can be reconciled. Although he held other prebends, Domesday Nigel was never called a clergyman, and he held secular lands as a tenant-in-chief of the king. On the other hand, Wistanstow Nigel was definitely a clerk and a personal physician who held his ecclesiastical benefice from the earl. Domesday Nigel evidently lived past 1100, but Wistanstow Nigel died before 1098. The records are frankly confusing, but it now seems possible that two physicians named Nigel were involved with the Wistanstow complex.

Other scholars have noted this contradictory evidence, but, wishing to emphasize the Domesday details, they dismissed the attribution of the position of doctor to the earl as a mistake in the records.[3] Such students invariably assumed that there were few Anglo-Norman doctors, but my own research has revealed a substantial number. Nigel of Domesday and Nigel of Wistanstow may both have been members of this large company. Wistanstow Nigel should probably have been listed among the physicians of 1066–1100, but a lingering doubt about his separate identity urges this more cautious placement.

---

[1]*Domesday Book*, 1:1v (Kent), 49v(Hampshire), 52, 64v, 65, 73 (Wiltshire), 91 (Somerset), 162v (Gloucester), 176, 183 (Hereford), 252, 252v, 260 (Shropshire); 4:2, 5, 7, 10, 13, 14, 17, 158 (Devon); 1:67, 180, 181, 483 (Somerset); Galbraith and Tait, eds., *Herefordshire Domesday*, pp. 4, 32, 34, 77, 91, 92; *V.C.H. Wiltshire*, 2:103; Talbot and Hammond, p. 232; Brett, *English Church*, p. 110.
[2]B.L., Additional 50121, fo. 51.
[3]Eyton, *Antiquities of Shropshire*, 1:209, 11:356, thought that Nigel was the earl's physician and that he was also Domesday Nigel. James Tait, in *V.C.H., Shropshire* 1:290, said that Earl

Roger's gift to his physician could not be reconciled with Domesday Nigel's tenancy-in-chief here and elsewhere. For him, Nigel was physician only to the Conqueror, not to Roger of Mont-gomery. Marjorie Chibnall, *V.C.H., Shropshire*, 2:71, noted that the patronage of the church belonged to the crown under the Confessor and then passed to Earl Roger, but she also believed that Nigel was the Conqueror's physician. Mason, "Norman Earls of Shropshire," p. 252, de-clared that Nigel's position as the earl's physician could simply be dismissed as an error, since in accepting him Eyton had failed to take the evidence from other shires into account, and that Nigel was only the Conqueror's physician, if anyone's.

52. NIGEL OF CALNE

Secular clerk in London and Salisbury; physician 1107/12–30 to bishop and to king; see Chapter 3.

53. OSMAR, MIDDLESEX

Osmar *medicus* held land at Harrow in Middlesex on a manor belonging to the archbishop of Canterbury. The physician apparently held one and one-half hides and rights of pannage for his animals at an annual rent of five shillings. He must have been dead by 1150x1152, at which time Archbishop Theobald made a charter for Ed-mund, the son of Osmar, the physician, confirming his right to his father's tenancy.[1]

[1]Saltman, *Theobald*, p. 345, no. 124. Not in Talbot and Hammond.

54. PAIN, WINCHESTER

In the Winchester survey of 1148, Pain *medicus* was listed as paying the bishop a rent of 12 pence for land outside Southgate.[1] Fellow practitioners William and Rich-ard were listed in the same survey as making more substantial payments.

[1]Barlow, ed., *Winton Domesday*, p. 138. Talbot and Hammond erroneously listed him as hav-ing lived in the eleventh century, p. 234.

55. PAULINUS, YORK

Paulinus was one of several physicians active in York. His long career suggests a gradual movement from personal consultant to a single baronial family or abbey to a more general practice in the city of York. Low ranking in witness lists implies that he was a layman. First mention of him is made before 1123x1133, when he attested a grant of Bernard de Balliol for Saint Mary's Abbey in York.[1] He also signed a later agreement of the same lord with Abbot Savaric.[2] Oddly, both documents have the same witnesses. A second charter of Savaric was also signed by the physician.[3] Gun-dreda de Gournay, wife of Nigel de Albini and mother of Roger de Mowbray, was a great patron of hospitals, as was her son. One of her grants to the poor of Saint Peter's Hospital was attested by Paulinus, "medicus of York."[4] An agreement made before the county court sitting in the cathedral crypt in 1166 was attested by eighteen men, including Paulinus *medicus*.[5] Abbot Clement of Saint Mary's also had Paulinus wit-ness two writs.[6] Paulinus's career and his involvement with Saint Mary's Abbey thus stretches from before 1133 until after 1166.

Paulinus, the doctor of York, has sometimes been confused with Master Paulinus, one of the sons of Bishop Ralph of Orkney. This Paulinus also appeared frequently in

Yorkshire records as witness to many charters. After 1164 he was given the rich ecclesiastical living of Leeds and was often called Paulinus of Leeds. He personally observed a series of miracles in York Minster in 1177, became master of Saint Peter's
Hospital after 1184, and was offered the bishopric of Carlisle in 1186 by Henry II,
but refused it. He died in 1201x1202.[7]

Paulinus was naturally a popular name in York since it commemorated the city's
first bishop (d. 644). It is thus sometimes impossible to distinguish in the records
whether Paulinus the doctor or Paulinus of Leeds was intended, or whether a completely different party was involved.[8]

[1]Napier and Stevenson, eds., *Crawford Collection*, pp. 34–35, no. 18 (with a suggested date of
1150); *E.Y.C.*, 1:439–40, no 561 (dated as 1132x1153). The date can now be fixed more precisely. In 1123x1133 King Henry confirmed the grants to Saint Mary's, as the charters of Guy de
Balliol testify. Guy's charter was for Abbot Richard (1113/14–18), and Bernard had succeeded
his uncle by 1130.
[2]Hodgson, *Northumberland*, 6:23 (dated 1138x1161, the rule of Abbot Savaric). The coincidence of witnesses and the nature of the agreement put this very early in Savaric's term. Bernard
died about 1167.
[3]*E.Y.C.*, 1:476, no. 606, (dated by editors c. 1140x1155).
[4]Dugdale, *Monasticon*, 7:609–10; Greenway, ed., *Charter of Mowbray* (dated by editor
1142x1154).
[5]*E.Y.C.*, 2:64, no. 718.
[6]*E.Y.C.*, 2:188, no. 848 (dated by editors 1161x1184, the years of Clement's term); *E.Y.C.*,
1:477, no. 607 (1161–84).
[7]Holmes, "Paulinus of Leeds." Paulinus's name appears in more than twenty deeds of the period. See also, Scammell, *Hugh du Puiset*, p. 10, n. 3. Talbot and Hammond seem to realize
that different men were involved, but the authors apparently think that each was a physician.
More confusingly, they cite the same evidence for three different individuals when there are in
fact only two men (only one of whom is a doctor), and when each has different documentation.
[8]For example, *Rievaulx Cartulary*, p. 513, no. 86, witnessed in 1160 by a Master Paulinus;
E.Y.C., 1:349, no. 450 (1143x1153) where a Paulinus attests at York with many others, including Bernard, the doctor.

56. PEDRO ALFONSO

Spanish layman, convert from Judaism, (1062–1142); famous author and scientist;
see Chapter 3.

57. PETER, BEDFORD

The nunnery of Harrold, in Bedfordshire, was founded in 1136x1138 by Samson le
Fort. Peter medicus was one of the witnesses to the foundation charter.[1]

[1]*Harrold Cartulary*, p. 16. Not in Talbot and Hammond.

58. PETER DE QUINCY, YORKSHIRE

Peter de Quincy becomes unusually vivid for a short period. Sometime before
1141, Alan, the earl of Brittany, Richmond, and Cornwall, wrote to Abbot Serlo of
Savigny, in Normandy, asking that several religious be sent to him in Yorkshire.
Serlo dispatched a party of one conversus and three monks, including the leader and
skilled physician, Peter de Quincy, apparently from Quincy in Yonne. They remained quietly with the earl and other northern magnates for several years.

Earl Alan, said to be a crafty man, was supposedly a supporter of King Stephen in the civil wars. He played, however, a rather ambiguous part in the royal rout at the battle of Lincoln. Perhaps to clear his reputation, Alan plotted to ambush the earl of Chester in revenge for the disgraceful capture of the king. The plan backfired and Alan himself was made prisoner, put into irons, and lodged in a filthy dungeon, where he became deathly ill. He was only delivered after surrendering some castles to Ranulf of Chester. Throughout Alan's ordeal Peter the physician remained by his side, tending his corporal and spiritual ills. The earl was very grateful and later described Peter as the "guardian of my body and soul."

After his release Alan became more concerned about good works. At some point he even claimed to have had visions. He rewarded Peter handsomely and urged his vassals to do likewise. For his part, Peter conceived the idea of establishing a new Savignac house in Yorkshire and went about the task with considerable gusto, perhaps with the aid of some local hermits. From Acris Fitz Bardulf he received a somewhat unsuitable site at Fors, in the North Riding, about 1143x1145. This gift was confirmed at different times by Alan, who evidently attended the raising of the first wooden church. There was also a grant to Peter from Roger de Mowbray, a champion of the nearby Savignac abbey of Byland.

Earl Alan visited Savigny when he was abroad and told Abbot Serlo about the new foundation begun not far from the earl's castle at Richmond. The abbot was anything but pleased. Savigny had experienced mixed success with its British plantations and had become very cautious about additional establishments. It was also in the process of moving closer to the Cistercians, with whose order it would soon merge. After Brother Peter had repeatedly written asking for an abbot and more monks, Serlo finally fired off a harsh reply charging him with having acted imprudently when he initiated such a venture without proper consultation. Despite the reprimand, Peter did not give up. Savigny was to hold a general chapter meeting of the congregation in 1146, and the physician, who was evidently a prolific correspondent, asked the abbot of Byland to take a letter to the conference so that those present could learn about his good works and regularize the status of his monastery.

At first Serlo vented his frustrations on the absent Peter, calling him rash, complaining that the new house lacked sufficient endowment, and recommending that the chapter close down the unauthorized creation and sequester its revenues. Like most deliberative bodies, the assembly of abbots stalled by appointing a board of inquiry to be chaired by the abbot of Quarr. This monk eventually visited Fors and put the issue to Peter and his three companions. They heatedly defended their achievement, boasting that they already had 5 ploughs, 40 cows, 16 mares, and 300 sheep, as well as many skins to tan and enough wax and oil to last two years. It was not enough, however, and sadly the little group opted for affiliation as a daughter house of Byland rather than endure complete absorption by Savigny. Abbot Roger of Byland then entrusted Peter with the management of the place and appointed one monk to set up a hostel and a conversus to run the tannery.

The subjection of the whole Savignac order to Cîteaux in 1147 gave new hope to the independence of Peter's foundation. In 1150 his house at Fors was dedicated to Saint Mary of Charity as a full-fledged abbey under John of Kinstan, a former monk of Byland, who brought along several other brothers of that house with him. Peter was made cellarer—not much of a reward for all his trouble. For a while the new abbey prospered, but severe rains in 1154 brought near starvation, and many monks urged a return to Byland. Peter was more resolute, and he set off for Brittany to seek the aid of Earl Conan, Alan's successor. That lord promised assistance, but unaccountably delayed forwarding it until 1156. When the aid finally came the whole community moved sixteen miles down the valley to a better location at Jervaulx in Wensleydale. (During their journey a man reportedly came out of his house, studied the moon and the stars, and declared that they were moving at a propitious time.) The abbey, now called Jervaulx, thrived, but relatively little is known of its subsequent history.

Peter also fades from sight, but he must have been an exciting character in his day. He certainly gives the impression of being a successful leader and a resourceful provider, and he never lost the loyalty of the original band from Savigny. Clearly he had a way with words, spoken and written, but his temperament leaned toward impetuous independence rather than docile obedience. His medical background is obscure, but there was another physician at Savigny from whom he could have received training. Peter's attendance on imprisoned Earl Alan was unselfish and effective. It has been suggested that the physician originally came to England to perfect his study of medicine, but this seems unlikely. However, he probably did have well developed artistic interests, for architectural motifs at Byland and Jervaulx show influences from his probable hometown, Quincy.[1]

[1] A good synthesis of these events is found in Auvry, *Congregation de Savigny*, 2:322–61. A medieval account of the first days of Jervaulx was recorded in a lost register from Byland Abbey, quoted by Dugdale, *Monasticon*, 5:569–74. For Earl Alan's characterization of Peter see Gale, ed., *Registrum Honoris de Richmond*, p. 99, no. 26. For the earl's capture in 1141, see *Gesta Stephani*, pp. 103, 117; and David, *King Stephen*, pp. 53–54. The land grants are in Dugdale, *Monasticon; E.Y.C.*, 4:23–26; and Greenway, ed., *Charters of Mowbray*, p. 125. For the puzzling remark about Peter seeking medical training in Britain, see Talbot, "Letter of Roger Abbot of Byland"; see also Cooke, "The Cistercians in England," who mistakenly overemphasizes a supposed Cistercian hostility toward medical practice. For the artistic parallels, see Peter J. Fergusson, "Notes on Two Cistercian Engraved Designs," *Speculum* 54(1979):15. Talbot and Hammond, p. 252–53.

59. PETER, CANTERBURY

Peter medicus attested at Canterbury in 1163 with his son John, who was also a physician. This is the first definite father-son medical team to come to light. Since John was a doctor in 1163, it is entirely reasonable to assume that his father had been an active practitioner at least twenty years earlier.[1]

[1] Urry, *Canterbury Under the Angevin Kings*, p. 97; see also pp. 110, 172, 234. Not in Talbot and Hammond.

60. PETER, LEICESTER

Peter, the clerk, was the physician of Robert de Beaumont, earl of Leicester (1118–68). About midway in his career Robert gave the tithes of Sopewich and Ringeston to his doctor, Peter.[1] This medicus also once held land beyond the Westgate of Leicester, which he later gave to Amigia, the wife of Roger of Wales, who subsequently gave it to Nuneaton Priory.[2] Before 1154 Peter was with Earl Robert when they both attested a grant of Duke Henry Plantagenet (c. 1153) for Haughmond Abbey.[3]

[1]Guery, *Historie d'abbaye de Lyre*, pp. 161, 569–70. Constable, *Monastic Tithes*, p. 110. Earl Robert subsequently gave the tithes to another of his clerics, Adam of Ely, and then to the abbey of Lyre. Thus Peter's gift would have come well before 1168.

[2]B.L., Additional Charter 47,599; Stenton, ed., *Danelaw*, p. 245. This was the only evidence noted by Talbot and Hammond (p. 423). The date of Peter's tenancy is not recorded, but Roger of Wales evidently made his gift to Nuneaton early in the reign of Henry II, c. 1155x1160.

[3]*Regesta*, 3, no. 379. Before 1163 Peter seems to have been succeeded as Robert of Leicester's doctor by a medicus named William, B.L., Additional Charter 48086.

61. PICOT, GLOUCESTER

Picot medicus seems to have been a member of the household of the earls of Gloucester. In 1147 he attested Earl Robert's foundation charter for Margam Abbey, and in 1166x1183 he attested a deed of Earl William.[1] The earls also had a chaplain named Picot who served from 1129x1130 to at least 1150x1159. He was probably the same man as the physician.[2] One of Picot the chaplain's benefices was the remote church of Saint Gundleus in Monmouthshire. Glastonbury Abbey had a small cell in the neighboring land of Basaleg, and in 1146 Picot and the Basaleg monks quarreled over their respective parish boundaries.[3]

[1]Patterson, ed. *Gloucester Charters*, pp. 14, 165–66. Not in Talbot and Hammond.

[2]Patterson, ed., *Gloucester Charters*, p. 13. The editor thought the chronology made it unlikely that Picot medicus (1147–1166x1183) was the same man as Picot chaplain (1129x1130–1150x1159), but it seems very probable to me. Several physicians had longer careers.

[3]Cowley, *Monastic Order in South Wales*, p. 167.

62. RAINIER, BERKSHIRE

Roger Mauduit and his wife Odelina came to the chapter of Abingdon Abbey and offered that monastery their land and houses in Oxford. They also gave 100 shillings, but the actual transfer of property was deferred during their lifetimes. This compact was made in the presence of Abbot Faritius and a number of laymen, including Rainier the medicus.[1]

[1]*Abingdon Chronicle*, 2:139. Not in Talbot and Hammond.

63. RALPH, EXETER

Ralph medicus was one of many witnesses to a charter of Bishop William Warelwast of Exeter (1107–37).[1] William was blind, and this may have been the reason he knew several physicians. Such disability did not prevent his traveling extensively, even making frequent trips to Rome as an envoy of King Henry.

[1]Napier and Stevenson, eds., *Crawford Charters*, pp. 29–30, no. 13. Not in Talbot and Hammond.

64. RALPH, LINCOLNSHIRE

During Henry II's reign Walter de Neville gave the nuns of Bullington a toft of land in Redbourne hundred, Lincolnshire, next to the toft of William, the son of Ralph medicus.[1] A more general confirmation of grants to Bullington by Reginald de Craci, made between 1150 and 1160, was attested by many people of the Redbourne hundred, including William Fitz Ralph.[2] Presumably, Doctor Ralph had already died. If William was twenty or more in 1150x1160, as seems reasonable, Ralph had surely been active about 1130x1140, or before. A William, son of Ralph, does account in 1130 for Northamptonshire lands of his father which Hugh de Areci then held in custody.[3] Members of the Areci family appear later with William Fitz Ralph.[4] It would therefore seem that Ralph medicus died before 1130, when his son was a minor.

[1]Stenton, *Danelaw*, p. 64, no. 98. A William, son of the physician, attests a deed of Hamelin, earl of Warren (1164x1185), *E.Y.C.*, 8:113, no. 68. He could be the son of this Ralph, or of Ralph of Beaumont, or of Hugh, the physician of Lewes.
[2]Stenton, *Danelaw*, pp. 61–62; also printed in Douglas and Greenaway, eds., *English Historical Documents*, 2:845. The name of William Fitz Ralph appears several times during the later twelfth century, e.g., *Danelaw*, pp. 79, 111, 213, 277. This Ralph medicus is not included in Talbot and Hammond.
[3]*31 Henry I*, p. 83.
[4]Stenton, *Danelaw*, p. 213.

65. RALPH, SAINT ALBANS

Abbot Geoffrey of Saint Albans (1119–46) came to an agreement with Edgar, the son of Earl Gospatric, about some land for the abbey. Among those who attested for the abbot was Ralph medicus, probably a monk.[1] Edgar was a sick man when he made the grant, and he may have come seeking treatment at the abbey from its physician, Ralph, and at the hospital of Saint Julian, founded by Abbot Geoffrey. His charter contains a special clause to the effect that when Edgar departed this life, his lands, as fully stocked as they were on the day he fell sick, should remain in the hands of the monks, despite any claim of his heir. Edgar may have expected that his death would be preceded by an expensive period of sickness during which his assets might be depleted; or, anticipating some mismanagement of his property if he fell ill, he may have wanted to insure that the monks would receive an undiminished gift.

Perhaps related to this distinctive deed was a transaction Edgar made with Tynemouth Priory about the church of Edlingham. The witness list is confusing, but the text mentions Abbot Lawrence of Westminster (c. 1158–73), who was a former monk of Saint Albans.[2]

Saint Albans later became quite a medical center. Before entering the monastery, two brothers from Cambridge, Matthew and Warin, studied at Salerno. From there they brought back two friends, Robert and Fabian, presumably doctors and probably Englishmen, who also entered the abbey.[3] Warin was prior before 1173 and abbot from 1183 to 1195. His successor, John de Cella (abbot 1195–1214), was called a second Galen in medicine. Fabian was subprior from 1214 to 1223 and donated three books to the abbey.

[1]Gibson, *History of the Monastery at Tynemouth*, 1:48, 2:21–2. In the English translation of the charter, four names, including that of Radulphus medicus, were omitted, but they were printed in the Latin version. Not in Talbot and Hammond.
[2]Ibid., 1:49. Master Ralph medicus, a royal clerk, was described as the physician of Abbot Lawrence and received from him the Oxford church of Bloxham for an annual rent of five marks; Westminster Abbey, Ms. Westminster Abbey Domesday, fo. 378. I owe this reference to the

kindness of Dr. Emma Mason of the University of London; see also Mayr-Harting, *Acts of the Bishops of Chichester*, p. 15. Rather than the Doctor Ralph known to Abbot Geoffrey, this man seems to be the royal physician, Ralph of Beaumont; see the following entry in this directory.
[3]Hunt, "Library of St. Albans," pp. 265–66.

66. *MASTER RALPH DE BEAUMONT, LINCOLNSHIRE*

Master Ralph de Beaumont was evidently the most prestigious physician in Britain since the time of Faritius and Grimbald. His early days are obscure, but later he became a wealthy landowner, a devoted bibliophile, a somewhat unscrupulous official, and a medical attendant for several great men, including King Henry II.

Master Ralph medicus attested at least ten deeds for Bishop Robert de Chesney of Lincoln (1148–66). Many fall toward the end of the episcopate, but others could conceivably be as early as 1148. It has been suggested that Ralph was a canon of Lincoln, but no prebend has been identified for him, and he never actually mentioned any clerical status.[1] His name appears in three other charters, two of which intimately concern Lincoln.[2] On numerous other occasions a plain Master Ralph attested Lincoln documents, and these designations probably also refer to Ralph, the physician. Moreover, possibly as early as 1150, Master Ralph medicus gave two nonmedical books to the Lincoln chapter library. Many of his cathedral associates were also donors.[3]

Ralph medicus showed up in pipe roll records from 1157 (the earliest surviving roll since 1130) to 1170. He accounted for lands in Derby, Essex, London, Nottingham, and Northampton (especially Barton and Gaitinton).[4] By 1166 he also held land in Lincoln.[5]

By at least 1157 Ralph the doctor was moving in important circles. In that year, at Bury and at Chichester, he was mentioned with Henry of Essex, the royal constable, and several others as being part of the great assembly that resolved a long-standing dispute between the bishop of Chichester and the abbot of Battle.[6] Less fortunately, he was also involved in some way in the extended litigation (1158–1163) called the Anstey case. After many delays, the plaintiff, Richard Anstey, was able to recover his estates. In an itemized record that he later prepared of his expenses, he noted that he gave Ralph, the king's physician, a total of thirty-six-and-one-half marks, evidently in different installments. What service or advice he received for this consideration—bribe may be too strong a word—is unclear.[7] It may not have been his only such commission, however. Sometime before 1177 Hugh de Oilli paid a Master Ralph, clerk of the lord king, perhaps our Ralph, fifteen silver marks for help in a land exchange.[8] Although the payments now seem irregular, there was nothing secretive or unusual about them at the time.

Ralph the physician was a member of the mighty Beaumont clan, which had immense power on both sides of the Channel and a long history of interest in medical affairs. His connection appears most clearly in the report of his tragic death. On March 3, 1170, one of the forty vessels that set sail with King Henry from Normandy for England was wrecked at sea. Among the lost were Henry de Agnis and his family, Gilbert de Sullney, and Master Ralph de Beaumont medicus.[9] In earlier days the name Ralph de Beaumont had appeared several times, but without his medical title. About 1118 he had been called upon to witness the foolhardy depredations of young Waleran de Beaumont, count of Meulan.[10] More than a generation later he was still attesting with the Meulans, this time with Count Robert II.[11] A plain Ralph de Beaumont paid a fine to the English exchequer about the same time and also attested a gift of Hamelin, earl of Warrene.[12] Master Ralph de Beaumont witnessed one of Henry II's writs at Newbury in 1162x1165.[13]

John of Salisbury wrote a rather odd letter to Master Ralph de Beaumont congratulating him on a stand he had taken. John noted that he found the position, which he never specified, uncharacteristic of a man who had formerly seemed to delight in courtly trifles and who had the mouth, but not the heart, of a philosopher.[14] It was hardly a flattering correspondence, but did suggest some basic change in Ralph's outlook, perhaps about the Becket controversy.

For a while Ralph medicus evidently also served as physician to Abbot Lawrence of Westminster (1158–75), who had formerly been associated with Durham, Saint Albans, and Lincoln. Ralph received the Oxfordshire church of Bloxham for an annual rent of five marks as a type of retainer fee.[15] This benefice had once belonged to Bishop Robert of Lincoln and would later pass to Seffrid II, the archdeacon and future bishop of Chichester.

It is remotely possible that more than one Ralph medicus was involved in all this activity, but the similarity of dates, places, and fellow witnesses argue against it.[16] Thus Master Ralph was a rather well-born practitioner, a constant traveler, and a physician who consorted chiefly with princes and prelates. He loved books and had the reputation of carefully feathering his own nest. Many people knew him, but he probably had few true friends.

[1]Greenway, in her edition of the Lincoln fasti, Le Neve's "Fasti," 3:135–36, lists and dates most of Ralph's attestations. The Walden Cartulary charter, B.L., Ms. 3697, fo. 43v, however, does not call him a clerk and can only be definitely dated 1152x1164, not 1160x1166. Ralph's appearances with Bishop Robert that are not mentioned in the Fasti include: Oseney Cartulary, 5:241 ((1163x1166); Ramsay Chronicle, p. 301 (1148x1160); and the Bardney Cartulary, B.L., Ms. Cotton Vespasian E 20, fos. 30v and 61v, where uncharacteristically he twice signed simply as Ralph medicus, omitting the word magister.

[2]Greenway, Le Neve;s "Fasti," 3:136, cites charters of Robert Mustela and William de Amundeville for Lincoln. Holdsworth, ed., Rufford Charters, 2:346–47, no. 685, notes a deed of Countess Alice and Earl Simon (c. 1160x1176) attested by a Radulpho medica [sic].

[3]This catalog of Master Hamo the Chancellor (1148–82) is published in Giraldus Cambrensis, Opera, ed. J. S. Brewer, J. F. Dimock, and G. F. Warner, (London, 1861–91), 7:170–71. Ralph wrote biblical commentaries on the Books of Kings and the Pauline Epistles. See also Woolley, Manuscripts of Lincoln Cathedral Library, p. viii. Master Ralph, clerk of Robert Bishop of Lincoln, attested with that prelate and Lawrence, the bishop's scribe; Red Book of Thorney, Cambridge University Library, Ms. 3021, fo. 421. Lawrence later became abbot of Westminster; see n. 15 below.

[4]Pipe Roll, 4 Henry II, p. 142; 5:4, 16; 7:31, 67, 8:8, 73; 9:36; 13:118, 119; 14:52; 15:76 (a fine for buildings he erected in the forest); 16:22, 17:45. In 1161 Ralph medicus received 14 shillings 3 pence, probably a medical fee, from the bishop of London; Hammond, "Incomes of Medieval English Doctors," citing Pipe Roll, 5 Henry II, p. 73.

[5]Red Book of the Exchequer, 1:382 (1166). He also accounted in Nottingham and Derby, 1:25 (1160x1161), 2:699 (1160–62); and Essex and Hereford 2:729 (1159x1170), 2:730 (1159x1170), 1:30 (1161–62).

[6]Palgrave, Collected Works, 7:27; Searle, Battle Abbey, pp. 33–34.

[7]Palgrave, Collected Works, 7:27–29; Barnes, "The Anstey Case." Richard of Anstey's principal adviser was a celebrated canon lawyer, Master Peter of Meldia, a member of the Lincoln Cathedral chapter; Greenway, ed., Le Neve's "Fasti," 3:133.

[8]B.L., Additional Charter 20462.

[9]Benedict of Peterborough, 1:4, Eyton, *Court and Itinerary of Henry II*, p. 135.
[10]Round, *Calendar of Documents*, p. 112 (1118x1131).
[11]*Beaumont Cartulary*, pp. 21 (1166, in Normandy) and 25 (1168, in Normandy).
[12]For amercements for land in Knaresborough; *E.Y.C.*, 1:391, no. 508; *Pipe Roll, 12 Henry II*, pp. 39–40. For Hamelin, *E.Y.C.*, 8:112, no. 68 (dated by the editor 1164x1185). If this is indeed Doctor Ralph, this charter must be redated to before 1170, and probably to before 1166 when he was in Normandy. A William, son of the physician, also attested the grant. Some other physician may have been his father, however, as several names intervene between this attestation and that of Ralph de Beaumont.
[13]*E.Y.C.*, 2:414, no. 1120.
[14]*John of Salisbury*, Vol. 2, pp. 338–41. I am grateful to Professor Brooke for this reference and an early copy of John's letter. He also cites a 1969 Ph.D. thesis from the University of Liverpool of J. Lally (which I have not seen) entitled "The Court and Household of King Henry II, 1154–89," which gives additional details on Ralph de Beaumont.
[15]Westminster Abbey, Ms. Westminster Abbey Domesday, fo. 378; Mayr-Harting, *Acts of the Bishops of Chichester*, p. 15; see also number 65, the entry for Ralph, the medicus of Saint Albans.
[16]Talbot and Hammond (pp. 260–61), with considerably less information, list five different Ralphs, whereas I think those men are all one individual. Since this section was prepared, D. M. Smith has edited *Episcopal Acta*. The attestations of Ralph medicus with Bishop Robert which are listed separately above are now in one convenient volume: nos. 72 (1148–66), 73 (1156–66), 112 (1160–66, as master Ralph phisico), 119 (1164–66), 161 (1160–66), 211 (1160–66), 226 (1148–60), 227 (1148–60), 244 (1148–66), 277 (1152–64). The clerk, Lawrence, attests seven of these same writs.

67. RAMELMUS

Monk at Much Wenlock in 1101; see Chapter 2.

68. RANULF

Former royal chaplain, became monk at Malpas before 1120; see Chapter 3.

69. RICHARD, WINCHESTER

Richard medicus was one of three physicians recorded in the Winchester survey of 1148. He paid the cathedral prior for land beyond Southgate.[1] Years later Richard medicus, perhaps the same man, held land in Seftwichene during the episcopate of Richard of Ilchester (1174–88), and also attested an agreement of that bishop in 1185 with the Hospitaller Knights whereby they assumed custody of the hospital of Saint Cross. A fellow witness with Master Richard medicus was Master Hamo medicus.[2]

[1]Barlow, ed., *Winton Domesday*, 1:139. Not in Talbot and Hammond.
[2]Holt, ed., *Pipe Roll of the Bishopric of Winchester*, p. 77, cited in Barlow, ed., *Winton Domesday*, 1:139. For the Saint Cross agreement, see Warner and Ellis, eds., *Facsimilies in the British Museum*, p. 67. A canon of Merton called Richard medicus attested in 1157x1161, but he was probably another man; see Saltman, *Theobald*, pp. 307–8.

70. ROBERT, WARWICK

Robert medicus, the son of Gregory, sold land worth four silver marks to Earl Roger of Warwick sometime between 1119 and 1153.[1]

[1]B.L., Additional Charter 21493. Not in Talbot and Hammond.

71. ROBERT, OXFORDSHIRE

Robert medicus, in company with Serlo medicus, attested one of Queen Adelaide's writs of 1136x1138.[1]

[1]*Oseney Cartulary*, 4:107, no. 75; Talbot and Hammond, p. 285.

72. ROBERT, YORKSHIRE

In 1130x1160 Orm, the son of Thor, gave land to the Austin canons of Nostell in Yorkshire in gratitude for having been cured by a Robert medicus. Property was also given to Robert, with the provision it would also eventually pass to Nostell if Robert lacked heirs. Talbot and Hammond thought Robert was probably a local leech of Nostell. He was, at any rate, evidently still a young man when rewarded by this grateful patient.[1]

[1]*E. Y. C.*, 3:324–25; Talbot and Hammond, p. 285.

73. ROBERT, YORK

Robert appeared with his fellow physician, Adam, to witness a grant for the hospital of Saint Peter's, York, sometime between 1143 and 1177.[1]

[1]See entry number 1, Master Adam, Yorkshire.

74. ROGER, LINCOLN

Roger medicus attested two writs of Bishop Robert de Chesney of Lincoln on October 1, 1151.[1] He signed last in a list of nine names. All the other signatories were canons and officials of Lincoln Cathedral. It has been suggested that Roger was probably also a canon, but no prebend has been identified for him.[2]

[1]B.L., Harley Charters, 84 C 47, 84 C 48. Not in Talbot and Hammond, Published in Smith, ed., *Episcopal Acta*, pp. 56–57, nos. 83, 84, from the Biddlesden Cartulary (B.L., Ms. 4714, fos. 2, 21). Smith evidently did not realize that the originals still exist. A Master Roger medicus, possibly the same man as Master Roger of Gloucester, attested a confirmation of William de Mandeville, earl of Essex, in 1167x1189; Elvey, ed., *Luffield Priory Charters*, 1:112, no. 119.
[2]Greenway, ed., *Le Neve's "Fasti,"* 3:143. A plain Master Roger attested with other Lincoln dignitaries in 1163; Smith, ed., *Episcopal Acta*, p. 95, no. 160.

75. MASTER ROGER OF GLOUCESTER

Master Roger medicus of Gloucester attested two deeds (1148x1163) of Gilbert of Monmouth and his wife Bertha to the Cistercians of Flaxley. The first grant, proceeds of a mill, commemorated the death of Earl Miles of Hereford (d. 1143) and was to be used for Mass wine and book repairs.[1] Roger must have considered himself identified particulary with Gloucester. A simple Master Roger, without medical title, sometimes appeared with members of the Monmouth family, and a plain Roger of Gloucester was also known in the area.[2] In its library Flaxley Abbey had a medical book written in English.[3]

[1]*Flaxley Cartulary*, pp. 133–34, nos. 6 and 7. Not in Talbot and Hammond.
[2]B.L., Additional Charter 20405 (1095x1100); published in Warner and Ellis, eds., *Facsimiles*

in the British Museum, no. 41; Dugdale, *Monasticon,* 4:596; *Regesta,* 2, no. 1041. Another appearance is recorded in *Bath Cartularies,* p. 55 (1122).
[3]Cheney, "Early Cistercian Libraries," p. 342.

76. ROLAND, CANTEBURY

Roland medicus attested a charter of Archbishop Ralph in 1120x1121. This would be after Ralph was partially paralyzed by a stroke.[1]

[1]Round, ed., *Ancient Charters,* pp. 16–17, no. 9. Talbot and Hammond, p. 316.

77. MASTER SERLO OF ARUNDEL

Secular clerk, physician to Queen Adeliza, 1136–60; see Chapter 3.

78. MASTER STEPHEN, LEICESTER

Master Stephen medicus was one of several doctors who associated with Robert, earl of Leicester. In 1148x1157 Stephen attested with the earl, his countess, and archdeacon Hugh regarding an agreement between the monks of Biddlesden and the canons of Saint Mary de Prato of Leicester.[1]

[1]B.L., Harley Charter 84 D 12. Not in Talbot and Hammond.

79. WALTER, KENILWORTH

Before 1143 Walter, calling himself clericus et medicus, attested a charter of Geoffrey de Clinton the younger for Prior Bernard of Kenilworth Priory.[1]

[1]B.L., Ms. Harley 3650 (Kenilworth Cartulary), p. 6. Talbot and Hammond list Walter as late twelfth century, but he was certainly earlier. Geoffrey is known from 1136; Bernard was prior from 1126 to 1148x1153; and another witness, William of Saint Barbara, became bishop of Durham in 1143. A "William son of the doctor" appears with one of Walter's patrons and may therefore have been Walter's son; *E.Y.C.,* 8:112–13.

80. MASTER WALTER, YORKSHIRE

Master Walter medicus attested a deed of Archbishop Thurstan of York and Reginald, the prior of Pontefract, in 1137x1140.[1]

[1]*E.Y.C.,* 3:163, no. 1470; *Pontefract Cartulary,* 1:61, no. 40. Talbot and Hammond, p. 363.

81. MASTER WALTER, NORFOLK

Master Walter medicus attested two baronial charters later copied in the Castle Acre Priory cartulary. One deed was composed for Robert of Pargrave, who is known to have flourished about 1148. The other, perhaps slightly later, transaction was for Constance, the wife of Ralph, son of Gosberchurche, and the daughter of Brian Scolland. Walter's relative (*conatus*) Master Fulk, also witnessed this. Since the Warrenne family was intimately connected with Castle Acre, this Master Walter could be the same man as the Walter medicus found with Adam de Ponyings.[1]

[1]B.L. Harley Ms. 2110, fos. 22v, 63; the second charter is published in Dugdale, *Monasticon*, 5:33. Not in Talbot and Hammond. A plain Master Walter attested another deed for Castle Acre; Neale, *Charters and Records of the Neales*, 1:127.

82. WALTER, LEWES

In 1146x1154 Adam de Ponyings made a declaration that the benefice his son Hamelin had been promised by the monks of Lewes had not yet been received. Until it was, he would continue to accept the substitute rents of three other churches. In the time of Earl Hamelin of Warrenne (1160–1202) Adam's other son, Adam, reviewed this agreement. Walter medicus witnessed both statements.[1] Also in Earl Hamelin's time the younger Adam attested with a William, son of the physician.[2] Evidently people thought the designation was so obvious tht they did not need to name the father. Since the Warrennes were deeply involved with Castle Acre, it is conceivable that this Walter medicus may have been the same man as Master Walter medicus from Norfolk, although it is odd that he omitted his title of master.

[1]Lewes *Cartulary*, 2:26, 60–61. Talbot and Hammond (p. 364) noted the first declaration only. [2]*E.Y.C.*, 8:113, no. 68. It has already been suggested that this might also be William, the son of Ralph medicus, or, since the last witness was Ralph de Beaumont, perhaps a son of that distinguished physician.

83. MASTER WALTER DANIEL, YORKSHIRE

Master Walter, the son of Daniel, was twenty-five years old when he entered the Cistercian abbey of Rievaulx in 1150. Nothing is known of his background, but his father, who entered the same monastery, may have been of knightly origin. Walter was a rather impulsive, contentious man, but he became a prolific writer of tracts on theology and friendship. Many of these works are now lost, but his biography of Abbot Ailred of Rievaulx (d. 1167) has been preserved, and it may have been his best effort. It paints a sympathetic picture of the saintly and sickly abbot whom Walter loved and treated for many years. It has been suggested that Walter was only the infirmarian of the abbey, but in a separate lamentation for Ailred he does refer to himself as a medicus. His discussions of disease usually exhibit a professional clinical detachment.[1]

[1]For Walter's life, see Powicke's introduction to Walter Daniel's *Life of Ailred* (Oxford: Oxford University Press, 1950), pp. xi–xxvii. Powicke cites a personal communication from Charles H. Talbot, ibid., p. xxvii, who offered the lamentation and thought Walter Daniel was an infirmarian. Powicke himself found the passage inconclusive. Walter Daniel and Abbot Ailred, both described as medici, were not included in Talbot and Hammond even though there is more concrete evidence for their medical practice than for that of most charter witnesses.

84. WILLIAM, LINCOLNSHIRE

In 1114 William medicus and his son Alan attested the charter that recorded the foundation by Alan de Credun and his wife Muriel of Freiston Priory in Lincolnshire as a dependency of Crowland Abbey.[1]

[1]*Calendar of Charter Rolls*, 3 (1300–26):102, an inspeximus of 1307. Talbot and Hammond, p. 373.

85. WILLIAM, BEDFORD

Before 1124 Countess Matilda, daughter of Countess Judith, gave to the nunnery that her mother had founded at Elstow in Bedford the land of William the medicus of Bourne End, Kempston (Burna). Sometime after she had become queen of Scotland in 1124, Matilda, her husband, King David, and their son Earl Henry confirmed the grant indicating that the land was worth twenty shillings annually.[1] King Henry of England confirmed her donation of the doctor's land too. [2]

Matilda also gave Elstow a mill and twelve acres and five virgates of land in Kempston, but it is not clear that these necessarily belonged to the physician. When King William of Scotland confirmed the grants to Elstow, the annual value of William the physician's land had evidently depreciated to four shillings, and only four virgates were mentioned. The mill was considered to be worth 100 shillings a year.[3]

[1]Queen Matilda died in 1130 or 1131; her original grant as countess seems lost but her confirmation as queen is calendared in Barrow, ed., *Regesta Regum Scottorum*, 1:166. Unlike the editor, I cannot see any reason to connect William, the physician of Kempston, with the William Peverells of Dover and/or Shropshire. See also Wigram, *Chronicles of Elstow*, pp. 15–23.
[2]Dugdale, *Monasticon*, 3:413, attributed this writ to Henry II, but the witnesses clearly belonged to the first Henry. Talbot and Hammond, (p. 373) accepted this incorrect date. *Regesta*, 2, no. 1654, 1828, corrects Dugdale's defective text and dates Henry's confirmation 1124x1133, probably 1130. A charter of Henry II, examined during the reign of Edward I, also values William's land at twenty shillings a year; Dugdale, *Monasticon*, 3:414.
[3]Barrow, ed., *Regesta Regum Scottorum*, 2:158, no. 55. There is certainly no reason to think that William, the physician, was still alive at this time.

86. WILLIAM, LINCOLNSHIRE

William medicus was included in a list of the townspeople of Revesby when William of Roumare, earl of Lincoln, established a Cistercian abbey there in 1143. Ailred, another medicus, was first abbot of Revesby from 1143 to 1147.[1]

[1]Stenton, *Facsimiles of Early Charters* pp. 1–3. Not in Talbot and Hammond.

87. WILLIAM, WINCHESTER

William medicus was one of three physicians mentioned in a 1148 survey of Winchester. He accounted a rent of thirty shillings to the bishop for lands outside Southgate.[1]

[1]Barlow, ed., *Winton Domesday*, 1:138. Talbot and Hammond, p. 373.

88. MASTER WILLIAM, CANTERBURY

Master William medicus attested two characters in 1148x1154 of Theobald, papal legate and archbishop of Canterbury, for Colne Priory, in Essex. A fellow witness was Thomas of London (Thomas Becket), who was then called a chaplain of Theobold.[1]

[1]*Colne Cartulary*, pp. 6–9, nos. 10, 15; Saltman, *Theobold*, pp. 301–2 where they are dated 1150x1154. Not in Talbot and Hammond.

89. WILLIAM, LONDON

William medicus was a canon of Saint Paul's Cathedral, London. He held the prebend of Sneating for a short time, between Ralph, the son of Ranulf Flambard, who last appeared in 1149 and Richard, the son of Nicholas, who first appeared in 1157x1162.[1] Evidently William had some business in Yorkshire, for he was present in 1154x1157 when Roger de Mowbray gave the tithe of the mills of South Cave to York Minister to increase the endowment of a prebend there. William was then called William medicus, canon of London.[2] He is also mentioned as a canon of London in a confirmation of this grant and some restorations by Master Robert of Saint Peter's Hospital issued by Archbishop Roger of York about the same time.[3]

[1]Greenway, ed., Le Neve's "Fasti," 1:77; not in Talbot and Hammond.
[2]Greenway, ed., Charters of Mowbray, pp. 209–10. I do not quite understand the dating 1154x1157. The gift could have been made before 1154.
[3]E.Y.C., 3:437, no. 1825; see also Greenway, ed., Charters of Mowbray, p. 210. Talbot and Hammond, p. 374, noted this and suggested that since Archbishop Roger of York was present, William may have been his physician. This seems very unlikely.

90. WULFRIC OF HASELBURY

Priest and hermit, important local figure in his area, c. 1080–1154; see Chapter 2.

APPENDIX II

A Register of Anglo-Norman Hospitals

Although I have been able to add a few hospitals and to redate several others, this register is essentially drawn from the magisterial volumes of the *Victoria History of the Counties of England* (*V.C.H.*) and the superlative catalog by David Knowles and R. Neville Hadcock, *Medieval Religious Houses: England and Wales* (New York and London: St. Martin's Press, 1971), hereafter referred to as *M.R.H.* The institutions on my list are grouped by counties, but only new or altered entries are supported by pertinent evidence.

BERKSHIRE

1. Abingdon, Saint John Baptist. For 6 poor men; founded by Abbot Vincent (1121–31); dependent on Abingdon Abbey (Benedictine).
2. Reading, Saint Mary Magdalene. For 12 lepers; founded by Abbot Anscher (1130–35); dependent on Reading Abbey (Benedictine).

BUCKINGHAMSHIRE

3. Aylesbury, Saint John Baptist. For lepers and the sick; founded in the time of Henry I by four townsmen: Robert Ilhale, William atte Hide, William Fitz Robert, and John Palnok.
4. Aylesbury, Saint Leonard. For lepers; founded in the time of Henry I by Samson Fitz William and Reginald Wauncy.

CAMBRIDGESHIRE

5. Anglesey, Saint Mary. Founded as a hospital in the time of Henry I; became an Austin priory 1212x1236.
6. Ely, Saint Mary Magdalene. For lepers; founded by Bishop Nigel of Ely (1133–69).
7. Sturbridge, Saint Mary Magdalene. For lepers; founded –1150.

CHESHIRE

8. Nantwich, Saint Nicholas. Founded c. 1087.

CORNWALL

9. Launceston, Saint Leonard. For lepers; founded –1075 by Count Brian of Brittany.

DERBYSHIRE

10. Alkmonkton, Saint Leonard. For leprous women; founded c. 1100 by Robert de Bakepuze.
11. Derby, Saint Helen. For the poor; formerly a house of Austin canons; became hospital after canons moved to Darley in 1146.
12. Derby, Saint James and Saint Anthony. Founded about the same time as the Cluniac priory of Saint James to which it was attached, c. 1140; Henry I aided one of the Derby hospitals.
13. Spital on the Peak, Saint Mary the Virgin. For the poor; founded in the early twelfth century.

DEVON

14. Exeter, Saint Mary Magdalene. For 13 lepers; founded c. 1092.

DURHAM

15. Durham, Saint Giles. For 13 poor sick persons; founded by Bishop Ranulf Flambard in 1112; in 1153 Bishop Hugh moved it to Kepier, closer to the river.
16. Durham, Saint Mary Magdalene. For 13 poor; founded –1152 (M.R.H., p. 357, said the hospital existed c. 1250, but Bishop William of Saint Barbara [1143–52] made a gift; Offler, ed., Durham Episcopal Charters, p. 170, no. 43.) Hospitals also existed at Bathel and at Sedgefield, both in Durham, in the time of Godric of Finchale (c. 1069–1170).

ESSEX

17. Colchester, Saint Mary Magdalene. For lepers; founded –1120 by Eudo Dapifer at the instance of Henry I; dependent on Colchester Abbey (Benedictine).
18. Ilford, Saint Mary. For 13 leprous brothers; founded c. 1140 by Adeliza, abbess of Barking.

19. Newport, Saint Mary and Saint Leonard. For lepers (?); mentioned 1156x1157; dependent on Saint Martin-le-Grand, London (secular canons).

GLOUCESTERSHIRE

20. Cirencester, Saint John Evangelist. For the poor; founded by Henry I; dependent on Cirencester Abbey (Austin).
21. Dudston, Saint Mary Magdalene. For 13 lepers; founded –1127; dependent on Llantony Priory (Austin).
22. Gloucester, Saint Margaret and Saint Sepulchre. For lepers; founded c. 1150; dependent on Gloucester Abbey (Benedictine).
23. Stow-on-the-Wold, Holy Trinity. For poor women; founded c. 1010 by Ailmar, earl of Devon and Cornwall.

HAMPSHIRE

24. Winchester, Saint Cross. For the poor; existed c. 927; founded perhaps by Saint Brinstan (d. 934); evidently later identified with Saint John's Hospital in the High Street (Barlow, ed., *Winton Domesday*, 1:329); there may also have been a second pre-Conquest hospital.
25. Winchester, name unknown, at the Westgate. Existed 1110; Herbert the Chamberlain was its patron (ibid., p. 52, no. 117; there was also a nearby hospice of 5 cottages for the poor, ibid., 1:49, no. 101; neither is in *M.R.H.*)
26. Winchester, Saint Mary Magdalene, 1½ miles east of city. For 9 leprous brothers and 9 leprous sisters; founded 1130x1148 by Bishop Henry of Winchester (*M.R.H.*, p. 404, said it was erected in 1158, but it was listed in the survey of 1148, Barlow, ed., *Winton Domesday*, p. 328, 90 no. 276, although not in the pipe roll of 1130.)
27. Winchester, Sisters' Hospital (Sustern Spital), outside King's Gate. For 21 sick; known in 1148, maybe 1110; dependent on cathedral priory (Benedictine) (*M.R.H.*, p. 337, suggests –1300, but see Barlow, ed., *Winton Domesday*, 1:328, 139.)
28. Winchester, Saint Cross. For 13 poor men; daily dinner for 100 others; founded 1132x1136 by Bishop Henry of Winchester; given to control of Hospitaller Knights in 1151.

HEREFORDSHIRE

29. Hereford, Saint Giles. For the poor and lepers; existed –1150; the round church suggests that it belonged to Hospitaller Knights (*M.R.H.*, p. 323, say 1158 +, but Cule, in "Early Welsh Hospitals in Wales," suggests –1150.)

HERTFORDSHIRE

30. Saint Albans, Hospital for Saint Julian. For lepers; founded by Abbot Gregory (1119–46) before 1145; dependent on Saint Albans Abbey (Benedictine).

KENT

31. Canterbury, Saint John, at the Northgate. For 30 infirm men and 30 infirm women; soon there were 100; founded by Archbishop Lanfranc –1086.

32. Canterbury, Saint Gregory, across from Saint John. For priests and clerks who worked at Saint John's and for retired clergy; founded by Archbishop Lanfranc –1086; became regular Austin priory about 1123.

33. Canterbury, Saint Lawrence. For 16 brothers and sisters; founded by Abbot Hugh in 1137; dependent on Saint Augustine's Abbey (Benedictine).

34. Chatham, Saint Bartholomew. For the sick; evidently founded by Bishop Gundulf (1077–1108); dependent on Rochester Cathedral Priory (Benedictine).

35. Dover, Saint Bartholomew. For 20 sick, lepers, and pilgrims; founded in 1141 by Osbern and Godwin, monks of Dover Priory (Benedictine).

36. Harbledown, Saint Nicholas, near Canterbury. For 60 lepers; soon there were 100; founded by Archbishop Lanfranc –1086.

37. Milton, Saint Mary the Virgin. For lepers; existing in 1155.

LEICESTER

38. Burton Lazars, Saint Mary the Virgin and Saint Lazarus. For 8 lepers; founded by Roger de Mowbray –1146 (*M.R.H.*, p. 349, says 1138x1162, probably 1147 + when Roger [d. 1162] went on crusade, but William de Albini gave it land –1146; ibid., p. 406.)

LINCOLNSHIRE

39. Eagle, name unknown. For sick and aged Knights Templar; founded –1136x 1148, perhaps by King Stephen, who granted manor to Bishop Alexander of Lincoln (another possible patron).

40. Elsham, Saint Mary and Saint Edmund. For the poor; founded c. 1130x1135 by Beatrice de Amundeville; managed by Austin canons.

41. Lincoln, Holy Innocents. For 10 lepers; founded by Bishop Remigius (d. 1092) or by Henry I.

42. Lincoln, Saint Sepulchre, Saint James, and Saint Catherine. For the poor and sick; founded by Bishop Robert Bloet (1094–1123); after 1148 Bishop Robert de Chesney gave it to the Gilbertine canons of Saint Catherine's Priory; Saint Catherine's Hospital was apparently a separate hospital at one time and later absorbed by Holy Sepulchre.

43. Partney, Saint Mary Magdalene. For the sick and aged; founded c. 1115, probably by Gilbert de Gant; dependent on Bardney Abbey (Benedictine).

MIDDLESEX

44. Holborn, outside London, Saint Giles-in-the-Fields. For 40 lepers; founded by Queen Matilda in 1101.

45. Holborn, outside London, Saint Andrew. Probably for the poor in Saint Andrew's parish; founded 1102x1103; dependent on the abbey of Cluny.

46. London, Clerkenwell, Saint John of Jerusalem. Perhaps mainly a hospice;

founded c. 1142 by Jordan Bricett and his wife Muriel; dependent on priory of Hospitaller Knights.

47. London, by the Tower, Saint Katherine. For 13 poor; founded by Stephen's queen, Matilda, in 1148; dependent on Holy Trinity Priory, Aldgate (Austin).

48. Smithfield, outside London, Saint Bartholomew. For the poor and sick; large hospital; founded by Rahere in 1123; dependent on Saint Bartholomew's Priory (Austin).

49. Westminister, Saint James. For 14 leprous maidens; founded –1100 by the citizens of London.

NORFOLK

50. Castle Acre. Founded by William of Huntingfield (d. 1155); dependent on Castle Acre Priory (Cluniac) (omitted from *M.R.H.*, but in *V.C.H.*, *Suffolk*, 2:87); Saint Bartholomew's hospital for lepers, at nearby Racheness, was founded in the time of Henry II, or before, by Herbert of South Acre, and was also dependent on Castle Acre Priory.

51. Hempton, Saint Stephen. Founded in the time of Henry I by Roger of Saint Martin and Richard Ward; Ward became an Austin canon and the hospital merely an Austin priory, but care for the sick was still maintained.

52. Horning, Saint James. For the poor and travelers; founded by Abbot Daniel (d. 1153); dependent on Saint Benet of Hulme Abbey (Benedictine).

53. King's Lynn, Saint John Baptist. Founded c. the time of Henry I; dependent on Benedictine priory in town.

54. King's Lynn, Saint Mary Magdalene. For 12 brothers and sisters, 3 of whom were sick or leprous; founded 1145 by Peter, the chaplain.

55. Norwich, Saint Paul. For 14 poor, aged men and women; founded –1093x1119 by prior and convent; dependent on cathedral priory (Benedictine).

56. Norwich, Saint Mary Magdalene, outside Magdalene Gate. For lepers; founded by Bishop Herbert Losinga (d. 1119).

57. Norwich, Saint Giles and Holy Trinity. For the poor; founded –1145 (*M.R.H.*, p. 381, says founded 1246, but there is a foundation charter for the hospital of Holy Trinity by Bishop Everard [1121–45] in Saunders, *First Register of Norwich Cathedral*, p. 63.)

58. Norwich, Brichtric's Hosptial. For poor women; known in 1144 (not in *M.R.H.*, but recorded in Thomas of Monmouth, *Saint William of Norwich* p. 148)

59. Norwich, Saint Mary and Saint John. For nuns (?); the church received a charter from King Stephen in 1136x1137 (not in *M.R.H.*, but see *H.R.H.*, p. 216, and *Regesta*, 3, no. 615); in 1146 two nuns from the hospital founded Carrow Nunnery.

60. Norwich, Saint Mary and Saint Clement. For lepers, the sick, and the poor; said to be founded by one of the first bishops of Norwich; there was another undated twelfth-century leper hospital, Horsham Saint Faith, dependent on Horsham Priory.

61. Thetford, Saints Mary and Julian. For poor travelers and pilgrims; founded in the time of Henry I; there was also an early but undated leper hospital of Saint John the Baptist, which later merged with Saint Mary Magdalene's lazaretto in

the thirteenth century; on the Suffolk side, Thetford had two other hospitals.

62. Wymondham, unnamed, near the bridge. For lepers; founded –1146 by William de Albini; evidently a cell of Burton lazars.

NORTHAMPTONSHIRE

63. Brackley, Saint James and Saint John Evangelist. For the poor; founded 1115x 1167 by Robert, earl of Leicester.

64. Northampton, Saints John Baptist and John Evangelist. For sick; founded c. 1140 by an archdeacon of Northampton (William?).

65. Northampton, Saint Leonard. For the sick and lepers; supposedly founded by William I.

66. Peterborough, Saint Leonard. For 13 lepers; founded –1125; dependent on Peterborough Abbey (Benedictine).

NORTHUMBERLAND

67. Hexham, Saint Giles. For about 8 sick and lepers of the area; founded c. 1114x1119 by an archbishop of York, probably Thurstan.

68. Mitford, Saint Leonard. For the poor; founded by William Bertram in the time of Henry I.

69. Morpeth, name unknown. For the sick; William de Merlay granted land to the infirmary house in 1145x1165 (M.R.H., p. 377, dated this c. 1160).

70. Newcastle-upon-Tyne, Saint Mary Magdalene. For lepers; founded by Henry I.

71. Newcastle-upon-Tyne, Saint Mary, Jesmond. For pilgrims (?); founded –1125.

NOTTINGHAMSHIRE

72. East Stoke (or Stoke-by-Neward), Saints Leonard and Anne. For the poor; founded –1125 by ancestors of the Lyndecortes.

73. Lenton, Saint Anthony. For 5 poor men; founded at same time as priory, c. 1102x1108; dependent on Holy Trinity Priory (Cluniac).

74. Newark, Saint Leonard. For lepers; founded by Bishop Alexander of Lincoln (1123–48), probably c. 1130x1135; had early connections with Saint Peter's York.

OXFORDSHIRE

75. Clattercotte, Saint Leonard's. For a maximum of 55 members of the Gilbertine order who had contracted leprosy; possibly founded by Bishop Robert de Chesney of Lincoln (1148–66); by 1260 it had become a regular Gilbertine priory.

76. Cold Norton, Saint Giles. For the poor (?); founded 1148x1158 by Avelina de Norton (d. 1158); dependent on priory Saint John Evangelist (Austin).

77. Crowmarsh, Saint Mary Magdalene. For lepers; founded –1142.

78. Oxford, Saint Bartholomew. For 12 leprous brothers; founded by Henry I –1129.

SHROPSHIRE

79. Bridgnorth, Saint James. For lepers; early endowments from Henry I, his clerk, Richard of Brecon, a certain Thomas the clerk, and Walter of Hengate (*M.R.H.*, p. 315, only said –1124, but see *V.C.H.*, *Salopshire*, 2:100).
80. Shrewsbury, Saint Giles. For the sick and poor; founded by Henry I; dependent on Shrewsbury Abbey (Benedictine).

SOMERSET

81. Bath, Holy Cross and Saint Mary Magdalene. For lepers; founded –1100 by Walter Hosate, sheriff of Wiltshire (d. c. 1113); later dependent on cathedral priory.

STAFFORDSHIRE

82. Lichfield, Saint John Baptist. Probably founded by Bishop Roger de Clinton (1129–48).

SUFFOLK

83. Bury Saint Edmunds, Saint Peter. For the sick, lepers, invalid priests, and others; founded by Abbot Anselm in the time of Henry I; dependent on abbey of Bury Saint Edmunds (Benedictine); the abbey also sponsored the leper hospital of Saint Petronilla, probably early in the century.
84. Thetford, Holy Sepulchre. Founded probably by William de Warenne II, earl of Surrey, c. 1139; dependent on Thetford Priory (Austin).
85. Thetford, Domus Dei. For the poor; may date from the time of William II.

SUSSEX

86. Battle, later dedicated to Saint Thomas Martyr. For pilgrims; known c. 1076; dependent on Battle Abbey (Benedictine).
87. Chichester, Saint James and Saint Mary Magdalene. For 8 lepers; probably founded by Queen Matilda –1118.
88. Lewes, Saint Nicholas. For the sick poor; founded by William de Warenne I (d. 1088); dependent on Lewes Priory (Cluniac).
89. Lewes, Hospitum. For pilgrims and travelers; founded in the early twelfth century; dependent on Lewes Priory (Cluniac).
90. Pynham, unnamed. At bridge crossing, probably a hospice for travelers; founded by Queen Adeliza, 1135x1151; dependent on priory of Saint Bartholomew (Austin).
91. Seaford, Saint Leonard (sometimes also called Saint James Hospital). For lepers; founded by Roger de Fraxineto –1147.

WARWICKSHIRE

92. Warwick, Saint Michael, Saltisford. For lepers; founded late in the time of Roger, earl of Warwick (1119/23–45).

93. Warwick, Saint Sepulchre. For pilgrims (?); begun by Henry of Newburgh, earl of Warwick (d. 1119/23), finished by his son Roger; originally belonged to canons of Holy Sepulchre.

WESTMORELAND

94. Scaltwaiterigg, or Kirkby in Kendal, Saint Leonard. For lepers; founded in early twelfth century.

WILTSHIRE

95. Wilton, Saint Giles. For lepers and the sick; founded by Queen Adeliza about 1135.

WORCESTERSHIRE

96. Worcester, Saint Oswald. For leprous monks; founded by Bishop Oswald c. 972.
97. Worcester, Saint Wulstan. For the poor and sick; founded by Bishop Wulstan c. 1085.

YORKSHIRE

98. Bagby, Spital. For the poor and sick; founded c. 1145 by Gundreda de Gournay; dependent on Saint Peter's Hospital, York.
99. Beverley, Saint Giles. Evidently founded by a certain Wulse –1066.
100. Bridlington, Saint Mary. Founded by prior and convent; Alan de Monceaux an early benefactor c. 1135; dependent on Bridlington Priory (Austin).
101. Broughton, Saint Mary Magdalene (near Malton). For poor; founded by Eustace Fitz John in 1154; dependent on Malton Priory (Gilbertine).
102. Flixton by Folkton, Carmen-Spitle, Saint Mary the Virgin and Saint Andrew. For 14 men and women, travelers; founded by Acehorn, a subordinate of King Athelstan, c. 940.
103. Goathland. For the poor; founded by the hermit Osmund, 1100x1109; Henry I a major benefactor; quickly became dependent of Whitby Abbey (Benedictine).
104. Malton (Wheelgate, New Malton), Saint Mary Magdalene and Saint Nicholas. Founded by Eustace Fitz John c. 1150; dependent on Malton Priory (Gilbertine).
105. Norton (by Malton), Saint Nicholas. For the sick and travelers, near bridge; probably founded by William of Flameville 1150x1169; aided by Roger of Flameville; dependent on Malton Priory (Gilbertine) (M.R.H., p. 381, says founded in 1189, but Roger died in 1169; see Greenway, ed., Charters of Mowbray, p. 132).
106. Otley. For lepers; near bridge; founded by Archbishop Thurstan of York (1114–40).
107. Pontefract, Saint Nicholas. For poor; founded c. –1066; about 1090 Robert de Lacy granted it to Cluiac priory of Pontefract.

108. Ripon, Saint John the Baptist. For the poor and travelers; founded by Archbishop Thomas of York (1109–14).
109. Ripon, Saint Mary Magdalene. For 18 lepers, blind priests, travelers; founded by Archbishop Thurstan (1114–40)
110. Upsall, in Cleveland, Saint Leonard. For lepers; founded –1146x1154.
111. Whitby, Saint Michael, Spital Bridge. For lepers; founded 1109 by Abbot William de Percy; dependent on Whitby Abbey (Benedictine).
112. York, Saint Nicholas. For lepers and the sick; a large hospital; founded by Abbot Stephen of Saint Mary's Abbey (1008–1112) or, less likely, by Abbot Savaric (1132–61).
113. York, Saint Peter. For the sick and poor; accommodations for 206 sick; founded 936 by King Athelestan; site moved under William Rufus; under Stephen began to be called Saint Leonard's; kings considered themselves special protectors of this large hospital.

List of Abbreviations

BIBLIOGRAPHY

The following sources offered information particularly relevant to this study. Original manuscripts, whether chronicles, treatises, charters, or cartulary collections, are listed by their current repositories. When possible, printed editions are cited by medieval authors. Publications of anonymous records are alphabetized by location.

MANUSCRIPTS

Cambridge. Cambridge University. Corpus Christi College Manuscript: 111.
_____. Gonville and Caius College Manuscript: 428.
_____. Jesus College Manuscripts: Q. D. 2.
_____. University Library Manuscripts: Ii. 4. 26, Ii. 6. 2, Additional 3021.
London. British Library. Additional Charters: 19573, 20405, 20462, 20465, 21493, 28331, 28347, 28353, 47381, 47599. Additional Manuscripts: 3697, 4714, 50121.
_____. Cotton Manuscripts: Claudius A VI, Claudius C IX, Faustina A IV, Nero A V, Vespasian E V, Vespasian E XX, Vespasian E XXV.
_____. Egerton Manuscripts: 3031, 3316.
_____. Harley Charters 45 C 32, 55 E 14, 83 C 40, 83 C 41, 84 C 47, 84 C 48, 84 D 12.
_____. Harley Manuscripts: 491, 1585, 1708, 2110, 3487, 3650, 3667.
_____. Landsdowne Manuscript: 939
_____. Sloan Manuscript: 2839.
London. Public Record Office. C 115/ K/ 6679; C 115/ K2/ 6683; E 132/2/13; E 164/22.
London. Westminster Abbey Muniment Room. Westminster Abbey Domesday.

Oxford. Oxford University. Bodleian Library Manuscripts: 479, Laud 247.
_____. Corpus Christi College Manuscript: 157.

PUBLISHED EDITIONS OF MEDIEVAL SOURCES

Certain entries are listed under their working titles.

Abingdon Chronicle—Joseph Stevenson, ed. *Chronicon Monasterii de Abingdon.* 2 vols. RS 2(1858).

Ailred of Rievaulx. *De Anima.* Edited by Charles H. Talbot. London, 1952.

Aldgate Cartulary—G. A. Hodgett, ed. *The Cartulary of Holy Trinity Aldgate.* London Record Society 7(1971).

Anglo-Saxon Chronicle—Cecily Clark, ed. *The Peterborough Chronicle.* Oxford: Oxford University Press, 1958.

Apuleius Barbarus—Robert T. Gunther, ed.. *The Herbal of Apuleius Barbarus.* Oxford: Roxburghe Club, 1925.

Bald's Leechbook—C. E. Wright, ed. Copenhagen: Early English Manuscripts in Facsimile, 1935.

Barlow, Frank; Biddle, Martin; von Feilitzen, Olof; and Keene, D. J., eds. *Winchester In the Early Middle Ages: An Edition and Discussion of the Winton Domesday.* Oxford: Oxford University Press, 1976.

Barrow, G.W.S., ed. *Regesta Regum Scottorum.* vol. 1 *The Acts of Malcolm IV (1153–1165),* Edinburgh, 1960; vol. 2 *The Acts of William I (1165–1214),* Edinburgh, 1971.

Bath Cartularies—William Hunt, ed. *Two Cartularies of the Priory of Saint Peter at Bath. Somerset Record Society* 7(1893).

Battle Chronicle—Eleanor Searle, ed. and trans. *The Chronicle of Battle Abbey.* Oxford: Oxford University Press, 1980.

Baudri of Bourgueil—Phyllis Abrahams, ed. *Les Oeuvres poetiques de Baudri de Bourgueil.* Paris, 1926.

Beaulieu Cartulary—René Merlet and Maurice Jusselen, eds. *Cartulaire de la léproserie de Grand Beaulieu de Chartres.* Chartres, 1909.

Beaumont Cartulary—Etienne Deville, ed. *Cartulaire de l'église de la Sainte Trinité de Beaumont-le-Roger.* Paris, 1912.

Benedict—E.G.R. Waters, ed. *The Anglo-Norman Voyage of St. Brendan by Benedict.* Oxford: Oxford University Press, 1928.

Benedict of Peterborough—William Stubbs, ed. *Gesta Regis Henrici Secundi.* 2 vols. RS 49(1867).

Bethell, Denis. "The Miracles of St. Ithamar." *Analecta Bollandiana* 89(1971): 430–31.

Birch, Walter de Gray. *Vita Haroldi.* London, 1885.

Blyth Cartulary—R. T. Timson, ed. *The Cartulary of Blyth Priory.* London: Historical Manuscripts Commission, 1973.

Botfield, Beriah, ed. *Catalogues of the Library of Druham Cathedral. Surtees Society Publications* 7(1838).

Boxgrove Cartulary—Lindsay Fleming, ed. *The Chartulary of Boxgrove Priory. Sussex Record Society Publications* 59(1960).

Bridlington Cartulary — William T. Lancaster, ed. *Abstracts of Charters and Other Documents Contained in the Chartulary of the Priory of Bridlington in the East Riding of the County of York.* Leeds, 1912.

Brinkburn Cartulary — William Page, ed., *Chartulary of Brinkburn Priory. Surtees Society Publications* 90(1893).

Brooke, Christopher. "Episcopal Charter for Wix Priory," In Patricia Barnes and C. F. Slade, *A Medieval Miscellany*, pp. 45–64.

Bruton and Montacute Cartularies — Two Cartularies of the Augustinian Priory of Bruton and the Cluniac Priory of Montacute. Somerset Record Society Publications 8(1894).

Calendar of Charter Rolls Preserved in the Public Record Office, vol. 2 (Henry III–Edward I, 1257–1300). London, 1906.

Carthew, George A. *The Hundred of Launditch and the Deanry of Brisley: Evidence and Notes from Public Records.* 3 vols. Norwich, 1877–79.

Chester Cartulary — James Tait, ed., *The Chartulary or Register of the Abbey of St. Werburg, Chester. Chetham Society Publications* 79(1920).

Chichester Cartulary — W. D. Peckham, ed. *The Chartulary of the High Church of Chichester. Sussex Record Society Publications* 46(1946).

Clark, Godfrey L. *Cartae et Alia Munimenta quae ad Dominum de Glamorganica Pertinent.* 6 vols. Cardiff, 1910.

Clerkenwell Cartulary — W. O. Hassall, ed. *Cartulary of St. Mary Clerkenwell. Royal Historical Society Publications,* 3d ser. 71(1949).

Cockayne, Oswald, ed. *Leechdoms, Wortcunning and Starcraft of Early England.* 3 vols. RS 35(1864–66).

Colne Cartulary — J. L. Fisher, ed. *Cartularium Prioratus de Colne. Essex Archaeological Society Occasional Papers* 1(1946).

Constitutio — Charles Johnson, ed. and trans. *Constitutio Domus Regis.* In *The Course of the Exchequer,* edited by Charles Johnson. London: Thomas Nelson, 1950.

Craster, Edmund. "The Miracles of Farne." *Publications of the Society of Antiquaries of Newcastle-Upon-Tyne* 4th ser. 29(1951):93–107.

_____ "The Miracles of St. Cuthbert at Farne." *Analecta Bollandiana* 70(1952):5–19.

Daniel, Walter. *The Life of Ailred of Rievaulx.* Edited and translated by Maurice Powicke. London: Thomas Nelson, 1951.

Davis, J. Conway. *The Cartae Antiquae, Rolls 11–20, Pipe Roll Society Publications,* n.s. 33(1960).

Dodwell, Barbara. *Charters of Norwich Cathedral Priory. Pipe Roll Society Publications,* n.s. 39(1974).

_____ "Some Charters Relating to the Honour of Bacton," In Barnes and Slade, *A Medieval Miscellany,* pp. 147–66.

Domesday Book — Abraham Farley and Harry Ellis, eds. *Domesday Book, seu Liber Censualis Wilhelmi Primi.* 4 vols. London, 1783–1816.

Dominic of Evesham — Michael Lapidge, ed. "Dominic of Evesham, *Vita S. Ecgwini Episcopi et Confessoris." Analecta Bollandiana* 96(1978):65–104.

Douglas, David C., ed. *Feudal Documents From the Abbey of Bury St. Edmunds.* London, 1932.

Douglas, David C., and Greenway, George W., eds. *English Historical Documents.* Vol. 2 (1042–1189). London: Eyre and Spottiswoode, 1953.

Downer, L. J., ed. and trans. *Leges Henrici Primi.* Oxford: Oxford University Press, 1972.

Dugdale, William. *Monasticon Anglicanum.* Edited by John Caley, Henry Ellis, and Bulkeley Bandinal. 6 vols. in 8 pts. London, 1817.

Eadmer. *The Life of St. Anselm, Archbishop of Canterbury.* Edited and translated by Richard W. Southern. London: Thomas Nelson, 1962.

Eadmer, *H. N.* — Martin Rule, ed. *Eadmeri Historia Novorum in Anglia.* RS 81(1884).

Edwards, Angela J. M. "An Early Twelfth-Century Account of the Translation of St. Milburga of Much Wenlock." *Transactions of the Shropshire Archaeological Society.* 59 pts. 2(1962–63):134–51.

Elvey, G. R., ed. *Luffield Priory Charters. Buckinghamshire Record Society* 15(1968), 22(1975); also in *Northamptonshire Record Society* 22(1968), 26(1975).

Evans, Joan, and Serjeantson, Mary S., eds. *English Medieval Lapidaries. Early English Text Society* 190(1960).

Evesham Chronicle — William D. Macray, ed. *Chronicon Abbatiae De Evesham Ad Annum 1418.* RS 29(1863).

E. Y. C. — William Farrer and Charles T. Clay. *Early Yorkshire Charters. Yorkshire Archaeological Society Record Series.* 12 vols. (1914–65).

Eynsham Cartulary — H. E. Salter, ed. *Oxford Historical Society Publications* 49(1907), 51(1908).

Eyton, Robert W. *The Antiquities of Shropshire.* 12 vols. London, 1853–60.

Farrer, William. *The Lancashire Pipe Rolls.* Liverpool, 1902.

Feet of Fines, 7 Richard I (1196). Pipe Roll Society Publications 17(1894).

Finn, R. W. *Domesday Studies: The "Liber Exoniensis."* London, 1964.

Flaxley Cartulary — A. W. Crawley-Boevey, ed. *The Cartulary of the Abbey of Flaxley in the County of Gloucester.* Exeter, 1887.

Foliot Charters — Adrian Morey and C.N.L. Brooke. *The Letters and Charters of Gilbert Foliot.* Cambridge: At the University Press, 1967.

Forbes, Alexander Penrose. "The Lives of S. Ninian and S. Kentigern." In his *The Historians of Scotland.* Edinburgh, 1874, 5:29–119, 159–242.

Fountains Cartulary — William T. Lancaster, ed., *Chartulary of the Cistercian Abbey of Fountains.* 2 vols. Leeds, 1915.

Fulbert of Chartres — Frederick Behrends, ed. *The Letters and Poems of Fulbert of Chartres.* Oxford: Oxford University Press, 1976.

Galbraith, V. H., and Tait, James, eds. *Herefordshire Domesday. Pipe Roll Society Publications* 63, n.s. 25(1947–48).

Gale, R., ed. *Registrum Honoris de Richmond.* London, 1722.

Geoffrey of Monmouth. *The History of the Kings of Britain.* Translated by Lewis Thorpe. Baltimore: Penguin Books, 1966.

Gerald of Wales — J. S. Brewer; J. F. Dimock; and G. F. Warner, eds. *Giraldus Cambrensis Opera.* 8 vols. RS 21(1861–91).

Gesta Stephani — K. R. Potter, ed. and trans. London: Thomas Nelson, 1955.

Gibbs, Marion, ed. *Early Charters of the Cathedral Church of St. Paul's, London. Royal Historical Society Publications.* 3d ser. 58(1939).

Gloucester Cartulary—W. H. Hart, ed. *Historia et Cartularium Monasterii Gloucestriae.* 3 vols. RS 33 1863–67.

Grainger, Francis, and Collingwood, W. G., eds. *The Register and Records of Holm Cultrum. Cumberland and Westmorland Antiquarian and Archaeological Society Record Series* 7(1929).

Gray, Arthur. *The Priory of Saint Radegund, Cambridge. Proceedings of the Cambridge Antiquarian Society*, 1898.

Greenway, Diana, ed. *Charters of the Honour of Mowbray, 1107–1191.* Oxford: British Academy, 1972.

Greenwell, William, ed. *Feodarium Prioratus Dunelmensis. Surtees Society Publications* 58(1872).

Guisboro Cartulary—William Brown, ed. *Cartularium Prioratus de Gyseburne. Surtees Society Publications* 86(1889), 89(1894).

Hardy, Thomas Duffus, ed. *Rotuli Chartarum in Turri Londoniensi Asservati.* London, 1837.

Harrold Cartulary—G. Herbert Fowler, ed. *Records of Harrold Priory. Bedfordshire Historical Record Society Publications* 17(1935).

Heales, A. *Records of Merton Priory.* London, 1898.

Henry of Huntingdon—Thomas Arnold, ed. *Henrici Huntendunensis Historia Anglorum.* RS 74(1879).

Hexham Cartulary—*Abstracts of the Cartulary of Hexham, Northumberland. Collectanea Typographica et Genealogica* 6(1840).

Historical Manuscripts Commission—*Reports of the Royal Commission on Historical Manuscripts.* London, 1870–.

Holdsworth, C. J., ed. *Rufford Charters. Thoroton Society Publications* 30(1974).

Holme Cartulary—J. R. West, ed. *St. Benet of Holme. 1020–1210. Norfolk Record Society Publications* 2(1932).

Holt, N. R., ed. *The Pipe Roll of the Bishopric of Winchester, 1210–1211.* Manchester, 1964.

Howald, E., and Sigerist, Henry E., eds. *Corpus Medicorum Latinorum.* no. 4. Leipzig and Berlin, 1927.

Hugh Candidus—W. T. Mellows, ed. *The Chronicle of Hugh Candidus.* Oxford: Oxford University Press, 1946.

Hugh the Chanter. *The History of the Church of York, 1066–1127.* Edited and translated by Charles Johnson. London: Thomas Nelson, 1961.

Hunter, Joseph. *Ecclesiastical Documents. Camden Society Publications* 8(1840).

Huntingdon Cartulary—William M. Noble, ed., *The Cartulary of Huntingdon. Transactions of the Cambridge and Huntingdon Archaeological Society* 4(1930).

Ivo of Chartres—L. Merlet, ed. *Lettres d'Ives de Chartres et d'autre personnage de son temps (1087–1130).* Paris: École des Chartres, 1855.

James, Montague Rhodes, ed. *The Bestiary.* Oxford: Roxburghe Club, 1928.

_____, ed. *Marvels of the East.* Oxford: Roxburghe Club, 1929.

Jeayes, Isaac H., ed. *A Descriptive Catalogue of the Charters and Muniments of the Gresley Family.* London, 1895.

John of Ford. *Wulfric of Haselbury.* Edited by Maurice Bell. *Somerset Record Society Publications* 48(1933).

John of Salisbury. *Metalogicon*. Translated by Daniel M. McGarry. Berkeley: University of California Press, 1955.

John of Salisbury—W. J. Millor. S. J.; H. E. Butler; and C.N.L. Brooke, eds. *The Letters of John of Salisbury*. vol. 1 (1153–61) London: Thomas Nelson, 1955. vol. 2 (1163–80) Oxford: Oxford University Press, 1979.

John of Worcester—John R. H. Weaver, ed., *The Chronicle of John of Worcester, 1118–1146* Oxford: Oxford University Press, 1908.

Kemp, Brian R. *Medieval Deeds of Bath and its District. Somerset Record Society Publications* 73(1974).

————, trans. "The Miracles of the Hand of St. James." *Berkshire Archaeological Journal* 65(1970):13.

Kirkstall Cartulary—William T. Lancaster and W. P. Baildon, eds. *The Coucher Book of the Cistercian Abbey of Kirkstall in the West Riding of the Country of York. Thoresby Society Publications* 8(1904).

Lacarra, Jośe M. "Documentos para el estudio de la reconquista y repoblacion del Valle del Ebro." In *Estudios de Edad Media de la Corona de Aragon*, edited by Jośe M. Lacarra. 2(Saragossa, 1946):469–574, 3(1947–48):499–727, 5(1952):511–668.

Lawrie, Archibald C., ed. *Early Scottish Charters prior to 1153*. Glasgow, 1905.

Lees, Beatrice. *Records of the Templars in England in the Twelfth Century*. London: British Academy, 1935.

Le Grand, Leon. *Statuts d'hôtels-dieu et de léproseries*. Paris, 1901.

Lewes Cartulary—L. F. Salzman, ed. *Cartulary of the Priory of St. Pancras of Lewes. Sussex Record Society Publications* 30(1932), 40(1934); J. H. Bullock, ed., *The Norfolk Portion of the Cartulary of St. Pancras of Lewes, Norfolk Record Society Publications* 12(1939).

Liber Eliensis—E. O. Blake, ed. *Royal Historical Society Publications*, 3d ser. 92(1962).

Liber Memorandum Ecclesie de Bernewelle. Edited by John Willis Clark. Cambridge: At the University Press, 1977.

Liber Monasterii de Hyda. Edited by Edward Edwards. RS 45(1866).

Liber Vitae: Register and Martyrology of New Minster and Hyde Abbey. London, 1892.

Loyd, Lewis C., and Stenton, Doris Mary, eds. *Sir Christopher Hatton's "Book of Seals."* Oxford: Oxford University Press, 1950.

Macer Floridus. Gotsa Frisk, ed. *A Middle English Translation of "Macer Floridus de Viribus Herbarum."* Upsala, 1949.

Mayr-Harting, Henry. *The Acts of the Bishops of Chichester, 1057–1207. Canterbury and York Society Publications* 56(1964).

Moore, Norman. *The Book of the Foundation of St. Bartholomew's in London. Early English Text Society* 163(1923).

Napier, A. S., and Stevenson, W. H., eds. *The Crawford Collection of Early Chapters and Documents*. Oxford: Oxford University Press, 1895.

Neale, J. A. *Charters and Records of the Neales of Beverley, Yate, and Corsham*. 2 vols. Warington, 1907.

Neugebauer, Otto, ed. *The Astronomical Tables of al-Khwarizimi*. Copenhagen, 1952.

Offler, H. S., ed. *Durham Episcopal Charters, 1071–1152. Surtees Society Publications* 179(1968).

Oliver, Arthur M., ed. *Early Deeds Relating to Newcastle-Upon-Tyne. Surtees Society Publications* 137(1924).

Oliver, George. *Monasticon Dioecesis Exoniensis: Records Illustrating the Ancient Foundations in Cornwall and Devon*. Exeter, 1846.

Orderic Vitalis—Marjorie Chibnall, ed. and trans. *The "Ecclesiastical History" of Orderic Vitalis*. 6 vols. Oxford: Oxford University Press, 1969–80.

Osbert of Clare—E. W. Williamson, ed. *The Letters of Osbert of Clare*. Oxford: Oxford University Press, 1929.

Oseney Cartulary—H. E. Salter, ed. *The Cartulary of Oseney Abbey. Oxford Historical Society Publications* 89(1929), 90(1930), 91(1931), 97(1934), 98(1935), 101(1936).

Paris, Matthew. *Chronica Majora*. Edited by H. R. Luard. RS 57(1874).

Patterson, Robert B., ed. *Earldom of Gloucester Charters*. Oxford: Oxford University Press, 1973.

Pedro Alfonso. *The "Disciplina Clericalis" of Petrus Alfonsi*. Edited by Eberhard Hermes, translated by P. R. Quarrie. Berkeley, Los Angeles, and London: University of California Press, 1977.

_____ *The Scholar's Guide*. Translated by Joseph Ramon Jones and John Esten Keller. Toronto: Pontifical Institute of Medieval Studies, 1969.

Peter the Venerable—Giles Constable, ed. *The Letters of Peter the Venerable*. 2 vols. Cambridge: Harvard University Press, 1967.

Pipe Roll, 31 Henry I—Joseph Hunter, ed. *Magnus Rotulus Scaccarii, vel Magnus Rotulus Pipae, Anno Tricesimo-primo Regni Henrici Primi. Pipe Roll Society Publications* 1(1833). (Other pipe rolls are cited by the monarch's name and year, e.g., 7 *Henry II*.)

Pont-Audemer Cartulary—Mesmin, Simone C. "The Leper Hospital of Saint Gilles de Pont-Audemer: An Edition of its Cartulary and an Examination of the Problem of Leprosy in the Twelfth and Early Thirteenth Centuries." Ph.D. thesis, University of Reading, 2 vols., May 1978.

Pontefract Cartulary—Richard Holmes, ed. *Chartulary of St. John of Pontefract (c. 1090–1258). Yorkshire Archaeological Society Record Series* 25(1899), 30(1902).

Poynton, E. M. "Charters Relating to the Priory of Sempringham." *Genealogist* n.s. 15(1899): 158–61, 221–27; 16(1900):76–83, 153–58, 223–28; 17(1901):29–35, 164–68, 238–39.

Prescott, J. E., ed. *The Register of Whetherel. Cumberland and Westmorland Antiquarian and Archaeological Society*, Cartulary Series 1(1897).

Rainald of Merton—Marvin L. Colker, ed. "The *Life of Guy of Merton* by Rainald of Merton." *Medieval Studies* 31(1969):250–61.

Raine, James. *The History and Antiquities of North Durham*. London, 1852.

Ramsay Cartulary—William Henry Hart and Ponsonby A. Lyons, eds. *Cartularium Monasterii de Rameseia*. 3 vols. RS 79(1884–94).

Ramsay Chronicle—W. Dunn Macray, ed. *Chronicon Abbatiae Rameseiensis*. RS 83(1886).

The Red Book of the Exchequer. Hubert Hall, ed. 3 vols. RS 99(1897).

Regesta, 1–4—*Regesta Regum Anglo-Normannorum*, Vol. 1, edited by H.W.C. Davis (Oxford, 1913); Vol. 2, edited by Charles Johnson and H. A. Cronne (Oxford, 1956); Vol. 3, edited by H. A. Cronne and R.H.C. Davis (Oxford, 1968); Vol. 4 (facsimiles), edited by H. A. Cronne and R.H.C. Davis (Oxford, 1969).

Reginald of Durham, *Cuthbert*—James Raine, ed. *Reginaldi Monachi Dunelmensis Libellus de Admirandus Beate Cuthberti Virtutibus. Surtees Society Publications* 4(1835).

Reginald of Durham, *Godric*—Joseph Stevenson, ed., *Libellus de Vita et Miraculis S. Godrici, Heremitae de Finchale, Auctore Reginaldo Monacho Dunelmensi. Surtees Society Publications* 20(1847).

Registrum Antiquissimum—Charles Wilmer Foster and Kathleen Major, eds. *The Registrum Antiquissimum of the Cathedral Church of Lincoln. Lincoln Record Society Publications* 27(1931), 28(1933), 29(1935), 32(1937), 34(1940), 41(1950), 46(1953), 51(1958), 62(1968).

Register of St. Osmund—W. H. Rich Jones, ed. *"Vetus Registrum Sarisberiense,"* or *"Registrum S. Osmundi Episcopi."* 2 vols. RS 78(1883–84).

Richard, Melville. *The Laws of Hywel Dda: "The Book of Blegywrd."* Liverpool, 1954.

Rievaulx Cartulary—John C. Atkinson, ed. *Cartularium Abbathiae De Rievalle Ordine Cisterciensis. Surtees Society Publications* 83(1889).

Ripon Cartulary—J. T. Fowler, ed. *Memorials of the Church of St. Peter and Wilfrid, Ripon. Surtees Society Publications* 74(1882), 78(1886), 81(1891), 115 (1908).

Roger of Howden—William Stubbs, ed., *Chronica Rogeri de Hovedene.* 4 vols. RS 51(1868–71).

Roger of Wendover. *Flowers of History.* Translated by J. A. Giles. London, 1849.

Round, John Horace, ed. *Ancient Charters, Royal and Private Prior to 1200. Pipe Roll Society Publications* 10(1888).

_____, ed. *Calendar of Documents Preserved in France Illustrative of the History of Great Britain and Ireland.* London, 1899.

Saint Albans' Chronicle—Henry T. Riley, ed., *Chronica Monasteri S. Albani,* 7 vols. in 12 pts. RS 28(1863–76).

Saint Bartholomew's Cartulary—Nellie J. M. Kerling, ed., *The Cartulary of Saint Bartholomew's Hospital.* London: Lund Humphries, 1973.

Saint Frideswide's Cartulary—Spencer Robert Wigram, ed., *The Cartulary of the Monastery of Saint Frideswide at Oxford. Oxford Historical Society Publications* 28(1895), 31(1896).

Saint Gregory's Cartulary—Audrey M. Woodcock, ed., *Cartulary of the Priory of Saint Gregory, Canterbury. Camden Society Publications,* 3d ser. 88(1956).

Saint Michael's Cartulary—P. L. Hull, ed., *Cartulary of St. Michael's Mount. Devon and Cornwall Record Society Publications,* n.s. 5(1962).

Salter, Herbert E. *Facsimiles of Early Charters in Oxford Muniment Rooms.* Oxford, 1929.

Saunders, H. W. *The First Register of Norwich Cathedral Priory. Norfolk Record Society Publications* 11(1939).

Sawley Cartulary—Joseph McNulty, ed. *The Cartulary of the Cistercian Abbey of St. Mary of Sallay (Sawley). Yorkshire Archaeological Society Record Series* 87(1933), 90(1934).

Sawyer, Peter, ed. *Textus Roffensis.* Copenhagen and Baltimore: Early English Manuscripts in Facsimile. 7(1957), 11(1962).

Selby Cartulary — J. T. Fowler, ed. *The Coucher Book of Selby. Yorkshire Archaeological and Topographical Record Series* 10(1891), 13(1893).

Shrewsbury Cartulary — Una Rees, ed. *The Cartulary of Shrewsbury Abbey.* 2 vols. Aberystwyth: National Library of Wales, 1975.

Slade, C. F. *The Leicestershire Survey of c.* A.D. *1130.* Occasional Papers of the History Department of the University College of Leicester, 1956.

Smith, D. M., ed. *Episcopal Acta.* vol. 1 (Lincoln Diocese: Part I, 1067–1185). Oxford for the British Academy, 1979.

Stenton, Frank Merry. *Documents Illustrative of the Social and Economic History of the Danelaw.* Oxford for the British Academy, 1920.

Stenton, Frank Merry, *Facsimiles of Early Charters from Northampton Collection. Northamptonshire Record Society Publications* 4(1930).

Stevenson, W. H. "A Calendar of the Records of the Corporation of Gloucester." In *Historical Manuscripts Commission, Twelfth Report.* Appendix 9. 426–27.

Summary Catalog of the Advocates Manuscripts, The National Library of Scotland. Edinburgh, 1971.

Talbot, Charles H., ed. and trans. *The Life of Christina of Markyate.* Oxford: Oxford University Press, 1959.

The Thame Cartulary. Edited by H. E. Salter. *Oxfordshire Record Society Publications* 25(1947), 26(1948).

Thomas of Monmouth. *The Life and Miracles of St. William of Norwich.* Edited and translated by Augustus Jessopp and Montague Rhodes James. Cambridge: At the University Press, 1896.

Tremblett, T. D. and Blakiston, Noel, eds. *Stogursey Charters. Somerset Record Society Publications* 61(1946).

Turner, G. J., and Salter, H. E., eds. *The Register of St. Augustine's Abbey Canterbury.* 2 vols. London, 1915, 1924.

Walberg, Emmanuel. *Le Bestiaire de Philippe de Thaun.* Lund: H. Moller, 1900.

Walker, David. "Charters of the Earldom of Hereford, 1095–1201." In *Camden Miscellany, no. 22. Camden Society Publications,* 4th ser. 1(1964): 1–78.

Warner, G. F., and Ellis, H. J. *Facsimiles of Royal and Other Charters in the British Museum, I(William I–Richard I).* London, 1903.

Webb, Edward A., ed. *The Book of the Foundation of the Church of St. Bartholomew, London.* Oxford: Oxford University Press, 1923.

_____.*The Records of St. Bartholomew's Priory and of the Church of St. Bartholomew the Great, West Smithfield.* Oxford: Oxford University Press, 1921.

Whitby Cartulary — John C. Atkinson, ed. *Cartularium Abbathiae de Whitby Ordinis S. Benedicte.* (1078–1547). *Surtees Society Publications* 69(1879), 72(1881).

Wigram, S. R. *Chronicles of the Abbey of Elstow.* London, 1885.

William of Malmesbury, *G. P.* — Nicholas E.S.A. Hamilton, ed. *Willelmi Malmesbiriensis Monachi de Gestis Pontificum Anglorum.* RS 52(1870).

William of Malmesbury, *G. P.* — William Stubbs, ed. *Willelmi Malmesbiriensis Monachi de Gestis Regum Anglorum.* 2 vols. RS 90(1887–89).

William of Malmesbury, *H. N.* — K. R. Potter, ed. and trans. *The "Historia Novella" of William of Malmesbury.* London: Thomas Nelson, 1955.

William of Malmesbury. *Vita Wulfstani.* Edited by R. R. Darlington. *Royal Historical Society Publications*, 3d ser. 30(1928). There is a translation by J. H. F. Peile, *William of Malmesbury's "Life of St. Wulstan."* Oxford: Oxford University Press, 1934.

William of Newburgh. *Historia Rerum Anglicarum.* Edited by Hans Claude Hamilton. 2 vols. London, 1856.

Winchester Cartulary—A. W. Goodman, ed. *Cartulary of Winchester Cathedral.* Winchester, 1927.

Worcester Cartulary—R. R. Darlington, ed. *The Cartulary of Worcester Cathedral Priory (Register I).* Pipe Roll Society Publications, n.s. 38(1968, for 1962–63).

Wright, Thomas. *Early Travels in Palestine* (London, 1848).

_____.*Popular Treatises on Science Written During the Middle Ages.* London, 1841.

MODERN STUDIES

Alexander, James W. "Herbert of Norwich, 1091–1119: Studies in the History of Norman England." *Studies in Medieval and Renaissance History* 6(1969):115–232.

Altschul, Michael. *Anglo-Norman England: A Bibliography.* Cambridge: At the University Press, 1969.

Amundsen, Darrel W. "Medieval Canon Law On Medical and Surgical Practice by the Clergy." *BHM* 52(1978):22–44.

Andrews, H. C. "The Twelfth-Century Charters of Reading Abbey." *Antiquaries Journal* 14(1934):9–12.

Appelby, J. T. *The Troubled Reign of King Stephen.* London: G. Bell and Sons, 1969.

Arbesmann, Ralph. "The Concept of 'Christus Medicus' in St. Augustine." *Traditio* 10(1954):1–28.

Auvry, Claude. *Histoire de la congregation de Savigny.* 3 vols. Rouen and Paris, 1896–98.

Baker, Timothy. *Medieval London.* London: Cassell and Co., 1970.

Baldwin, John W. *Masters, Princes, and Merchants: The Social Views of Peter the Chanter and His Circle.* Princeton, N.J.: Princeton University Press, 1970.

_____, and Hollister, C. Warren. "The Rise of Administrative Kingship: Henry I and Philip Augustus." *AHR* 83(1978):867–905.

Bannister, Arthur T. *A Descriptive Catalogue of the Manuscripts in Hereford Cathedral Library.* Hereford, 1927.

Barfield, S. "Lord Fingall's Cartulary of Reading Abbey." *EHR* 3(1888):113–25.

Barlow, Frank. *Edward the Confessor.* Berkeley and Los Angeles: University of California Press, 1970.

_____. *The English Church, 1066–1154.* London and New York: Longmans, 1979.

_____. "The King's Evil." *EHR* 95(1980):3–27.

Barnes, Patricia. "The Anstey Case." In Barnes and Slade, *A Medieval Miscellany*, pp. 1–24.

_____, and Slade, C. F., eds. *A Medieval Miscellany for Doris Mary Stenton.* Publications of the Pipe Roll Society, n.s. 36(1960).

Bartlett, S. E., "The Leper Hospitals of St. Margaret and St. Mary Magdalene by Gloucester." *Trans. Bris. and Glouc. Archaeo. Soc.* 20(1895–97):126–37.

Bateson, Edward. *The History of Northumberland.* 2 vols. Newcastle, 1895.

Beddie, James Stewart. "Libraries in the Twelfth Century: Their Catalogs and Contents." In *Anniversary Essays in Medieval History by Students of Charles Homer Haskins*, edited by C. H. Taylor and John La Monte, pp. 1–23. Boston, 1929.

Bethell, Denis. "The Making of a Twelfth-Century Relic Collection." *Studies in Church History* 8(1972):61–72.

_____. "Richard of Belemis and the Foundation of St. Osyth's." *Trans. Essex Essex Archaeo. Soc.*, 3d ser. 2(1970):299–327.

_____. "William of Corbeil and the Canterbury-York Dispute," *JEH* 19(1968):145–59.

Bishop, Edmund. *Liturgica Historica.* Oxford: Oxford University Press, 1918.

Bishop, T.A.M. *Scriptores Regis.* Oxford: Oxford University Press, 1961.

Blake, D. W. "Bishop William Warelwast." *Transactions of the Devonshire Association for the Advancement of Science, Literature, and Art* 104(1972):15–33.

Bloch, Marc. *Les Rois thaumaturges.* Strasburg, 1924. Translated by J. E. Anderson. *The Royal Touch.* London: Routledge and Kegan Paul, 1973.

Bloom, J. Harvey. "An Introduction to the Cartulary of St. Mary's Warwick." *Trans. Bris. Glouc. Archaeo. Soc.* 37(1914):79–91.

Bonser, Wilfrid. *The Medical Background of Anglo-Saxon England.* London, 1963.

_____. "Epidemics During the Anglo-Saxon Period." *Journal of the British Archaeological Association*, 3d ser. 9(1944):48–71.

Blunt, Wilfrid, and Raphael, Sandra. *The Illustrated Herbal.* London: Frances Lincoln Publishers, in association with George Weidenfeld and Nicolson, 1979.

Brett, Martin. *The English Church Under Henry I.* Oxford: Oxford University Press, 1975.

Brooke, Christopher. "Gregorian Reform in Action: Clerical Marriage in England, 1050–1200." *Cambridge Historical Journal* 12(1956):1–21.

_____. "The Missionary at Home: The Church in the Towns, 1000–1250." *Studies in Church History* 4(1970):59–83.

_____. "St. Peter of Gloucester and St. Cadoc of Llancarfan." In *Celt and Saxon*, edited by Nora K. Chadwick, pp. 258–322. Cambridge: At the University Press, 1963.

_____. Keir, Gillian. *London, 800–1216: The Shaping of a City.* Berkely and Los Angeles: University of California Press, 1975.

Brooks, F. W. "The Hospital of the Holy Innocents Without Lincoln." *Associated Architectural Societies, Reports and Papers* 42 (1937):157–88.

Brown, David. *Anglo-Saxon England.* Totowa, N.J.: Rowman and Littlefield, 1978.

Bullough, Vern L. *The Development of Medicine as a Profession.* New York: Hofner Publishing Co., 1966.

_____. "Medieval Medical and Scientific Views of Women." *Viator* 4(1973):485–501.

Bynum, Caroline W. "The Spirituality of Regular Canons in the Twelfth Century: A New Approach." *Medievalia et Humanistica* 4(1973): 3–24.

Cheney, C. R. *Episcopal Visitations of Monasteries in the Thirteenth Century.* Manchester, 1931.

_____. *English Bishops' Chanceries, 1100–1250*. Manchester 1950.

_____. "English Cistercian Libraries: The First Century." In his *Medieval Texts and Studies*, pp. 328–45. Oxford. Oxford University Press, 1973.

Chibnall, Margorie. "Monks and Pastoral Work." *JEH* 18(1967): 165–72.

Clagett, Marshall. "The Medieval Latin Translations from the Arabic Elements of Euclid, with Special Emphasis on the Versions of Adelard of Bath." *Isis* 44(1953): 16–42.

_____. "Adelard of Bath." *Dictionary of Scientific Biography*. 1:61–64.

Clanchy, M. T. "Moderni in Education and Government in England." *Speculum* 50 (1975):671–88.

Clark, John Willis. *The Observers in Use at the Augustinian Priory of St. Giles and Andrew at Barnwell, Cambridge*. Cambridge, 1897.

Clarke, Basil. *Mental Disorders in Earlier Britain: Exploratory Studies*. Cardiff: University of Wales Press, 1975.

Clay, C. T. "Early Precentors and Chancellors of York." *Yorkshire Archaelogical Journal* 35(1940–43):116–38.

_____. "The Family of Amundeville." *Lincolnshire Architectural and Archaeological Society, Reports and Papers*, n.s. 3(1948):109–36.

Clay, Rotha Mary. *The Medieval Hospitals of England*. London: Methuen, 1909.

Clerval, A. *Les Écoles de Chartres au moyen age*. Paris, 1895.

Collingwood, Robin I., and Richmond, Ian. *The Archaelogy of Roman Britain*. London: Methuen, 1969.

Constable, Giles. *Monastic Tithes From Their Origins to the Twelfth Century*. Cambridge: 1964.

Cooke, Alice M. "The Settlement of the Cistercians in England." *EHR* 8 (1893):625–76.

Corner, George W. "On Early Salernitan Surgery and Especially the 'Bamberg Surgery'." *BHM* 5(1937):1–32.

_____. "Salernitan Surgery in the Twelfth Century." *British Journal of Surgery* 25 (1937):84–99.

Coulton, G. G. *Social Life in Britain from the Conquest to the Reformation*. Cambrige, 1918.

Cowley, F. G. *The Monastic Order in South Wales, 1066–1349*. Cardiff: University of Wales Press, 1977.

Creighton, Charles. *History of Epidemics in Britain*. 2 vols. 1891–94. London, 1965.

Cronin, Grover, Jr. "The Bestiary and the Medieval Mind: Some Complexities." *Modern Language Quarterly* 2(1941):191–98.

Cronne, H. A. "An Agreement Between Simon, bishop of Worcester, and Waleran, earl of Worcester." *University of Birmingham Historical Journal* 2(1949–50):201–7.

_____. *The Reign of King Stephen: Anarchy in England, 1135–1154*. London: Weidenfeld and Nicholson, 1970.

Cule, John. "The Court Mediciner and Medicine in the Laws of Wales." *JHM* 21 (1966):213–36.

_____. "Some Early Hospitals in Wales and the Border." *National Library of Wales Journal* 20(1977):97–130.

Cunliffe, Barry. *Roman Bath Discovered*. London: Routledge and Kegan Paul, 1971.

Curley, Michael J. *Physiologus*. Austin and London: University of Texas Press, 1979.

Dainton, Courtney. *The Story of England's Hospitals*. London, 1961.

Darby, H. C., and Finn, R. Weldon. *The Domesday Geography of South West England*. Cambridge: At the University Press, 1962.

_____, and Maxwell, I. S. *The Domesday Geography of Northern England*. Cambridge: At the University Press, 1962.

_____, and Terett, I. B. *The Domesday Geography of Midland England*. Cambridge: At the University Press, 1971.

Davis, G.R.C. *Medieval Cartularies of Great Britain: A Short Catalogue*. London, 1958.

Davis, H.W.C. "Henry of Blois and Brian Fitz Count." *EHR* 25(1910):297–303.

_____. "London Lands and Liberties of St. Paul's, 1066–1135." In *Essays in Medieval History Presented to Thomas Frederick Tout*, edited by A. G. Little and F. M. Powicke, Manchester, 1925.

Davis, R.H.C. *King Stephen, 1135–1154*. 2d. ed. London: Longmans, 1977.

_____. "Monks of St. Edmunds, 1021–1148. *History* 40(1955):227–239.

Demaitre, Luke. "Theory and Practice in Medical Education at the University of Montpellier in the Thirteenth and Fourteenth Centuries." *JHM* 30(1975):103–23.

Dereene, C. "Les Coutumes de Saint Quentin de Beauvais et de Springiersback." *Revue d'histoire ecclesiastique* 43(1948):411–12.

Dick, Hugh G. "Students of Physics and Astrology." *JHM* 1(1946):300–15, 419–33.

Dickinson, John C. *The Origins of the Austin Canons and Their Introduction into England*. London, 1950.

_____. "English Regular Canons and the Continent in the Twelfth Century." *Trans. Royal Hist. Soc.*, 5th ser. 1(1951):71–89.

Douglas, David C. *The Social Structure of Medieval East Anglia*. Oxford, 1927.

_____. *William the Conqueror: The Norman Impact upon England*. Berkeley and Los Angeles: University of California Press, 1964.

Druce, George R. "The Caladrius and its Legend, Sculpted Upon the Twelfth-Century Doorway of Alne Church, Yorkshire." *Archaeological Journal* 69(1912): 381–416.

_____. "The Medieval Bestiaries and Their Influence on Ecclesiastical Decorative Art." *Journal of the British Archaeological Association*, n.s. 25(1919):41–82, 26(1920):35–79.

Durbreuil-Chambardel, Louis. *Les médecins dans l'ouest de la France aux XIe et XIIe siècles*. Paris: Société française d'histoire de la médecine, 1914.

Dunlop, D. M. "Arabic Medicine in England." *JHM* 11(1956):166–82.

Dyson, A. G. "The Monastic Patronage of Bishop Alexander of Lincoln." *JEH* 26 (1975):1–24.

Ellis, May Heane. "The Bridges of Gloucester and the Hospital between the Bridges." *Trans. Bris. and Glouc. Archaeo. Soc.* 51(1929):169–210.

Engbring, Gertrude. "Saint Hildegard, Twelfth-Century Physician." *BHM* 8(1940): 770–84.

Engels, L. J. " 'De obitu Willelmi ducis Normannorum regisque Anglorum': Texte, modèles, valeur, et origine." In *Mélanges Christine Mohrmann*. pp. 240–42. Utrecht and Angers, 1973.

Evans, Gillian R. "Difficillima et Ardua: Theory and Practice in Treaties on the Abacus, 950–1150." *Journal of Medieval History* 3(1977):21–38.

―――――. "From Abacus to Algorism: Theory and Practice in Medieval Arithmatic." *British Journal for the History of Science* 10(1977):114–31.

―――――. "Schools and Scholars: The Study of the Abacus in English Schools, c. 980–1150." *EHR* 94(1979):71–89.

Eyton, Robert W. *Court, Household, and Itinerary of King Henry II*. London, 1878.

―――――. *Domesday Studies: An Analysis and Digest of the Somerset Survey*. 2 vols. London, 1880.

Farmer, David Hugh. *The Oxford Dictionary of Saints*. Oxford: Oxford University Press, 1978.

―――――. "William of Malmesbury's Life and Works." *JEH* 13(1962):39–54.

Farrer, William. *Honors and Knights, Fees*. 3 vols. London, 1923–25.

Fergusson, Peter J. "Notes on Two Cistercian Engraved Designs." *Speculum* 54(1979):1–17.

Finucane, Ronald C. *Miracles and Pilgrims: Popular Beliefs in Medieval England*. London: J. M. Dent and Sons, 1977.

Flint, Valerie I. J. "The Career of Honorius Augustodunensis: Some Fresh Evidence." *Revue Bénédictine* 82(1972):63–86.

―――――. "The Chronology of the Works of Honorius Augustodunensis." *Revue Bénédictine* 82(1972):215–42.

―――――. "The Commentaries of Honorius Augustodunensis on the 'Song of Songs'." *Revue Bénédictine* 84(1972):196–211.

―――――. "The Date of the Chronicle of 'Florence' of Worcester." *Revue Bénédictine* 86(1976):115–19.

―――――. "The *Elucidarius* of Honorius Augustodunensis and Reform in Late Eleventh-Century England." *Revue Bénédictine* 85(1975):178–89.

―――――. "The Place and Purpose of the Works of Honorius Augustodunensis." *Revue Bénédictine* 87(1977):97–127.

―――――. "The Sources of the *Elucidarius* of Honorius Augustodunensis." *Revue Bénédictine* 85(1975):190–98.

Flood, Bruce P. "Pliny and the Medieval 'Macer' Medical Text." *JHM* 32(1977):395–402.

Forbes, Thomas R. "Medical Lore in the Bestiaries." *Medical History* 12(1968):245–53.

Forder, Anthony. *Penelope Hall's Social Services of England and Wales*. 6th ed. London, 1963.

Friend, A. C. "The Proverbs of Serlo of Wilton." *Medieval Studies* 16(1954):179–218.

―――――. "Serlo of Wilton." *Bulletin du Cange* 24(1954):85–110.

Gerould, Gordon Hall. "King Arthur and Politics." *Speculum* 2(1927):33–51.

Gibson, Margaret. *Lanfranc of Bec*. Oxford: Oxford University Press, 1978.

Gibson, William Sidney. *History of the Monastery Founded at Tynemouth in the Diocese of Durham*. 2 vols. London: 1846.

Godfrey, Walter. "Some Medieval Hospitals of East Kent." *Archaeological Journal* 86 (1929):99–110.

Golb, Norman. "The Forgotten Jewish History of Medieval Rouen." *Archaeology* 30 (1977):254–63.

Grabois, Aryeh. "The *Herbraica Veritas* and Jewish-Christina Intellectual Relations in the Twelfth Century." *Speculum* 50(1975):613–34.

Graham, Rose. "Four Alien Priories in Monmouthshire." *Journal of the British Archaeological Association* 35 (1929–30):102–21.

Gransden, Antonio. *Historical Writing in England, c. 550–1307* Ithaca: Cornell University Press, 1974.

————. "Realistic Observation in Twelfth-Century England." *Speculum* 47(1972): 29–51.

Graves, Edgar. *A Bibliography of English History to 1485*. Oxford: Oxford University Press, 1975.

Greenway, Diana E. *John Le Neve's "Fasti Ecclesiae Anglicanae," 1066–1300.* vol. 1 (St. Paul's London), London: Institute of Historical Research, 1968. vol. 2 (Monastic Cathedrals), 1971. vol. 3 (Lincoln), 1977.

Grendon, F. "The Anglo-Saxon Charms." *Journal of American Folklore* 22(1909): 105–237.

Guery, Charles. *Histoire l'abbaye de Lyre*. Evreux, 1917.

Gunther, Robert T. *Early Science in Oxford*. 1925. Reprint. London, 1968.

Hammond, E. A. "Incomes of Medieval English Doctors," *JHM* 15(1960):154–69.

————. "Physicians in Medieval English Religious Houses." *BHM* 32(1958):105–20.

————. "The Westminster Abbey Infirmarers' Rolls as a Source of Medical History." *BHM* 39(1965):261–76.

Hardy, Thomas Duffus. *Descriptive Catalogue of Materials Relating to the History of Great Britain and Ireland*, 3 vols. in 4 pts. RS 26 (1862–71).

Hart, Cyril. "The Ramsay Computus." *EHR* 85(1970):29–44.

Harvey, John. *English Medieval Architects: A Biographical Dictionary down to 1550*. Boston, 1954.

Harvey, Sally P. "Domesday Book and Anglo-Norman Governance." *Trans. Royal Hist. Soc.*, 5th ser. 25(1975):175–93.

Haskins, Charles Homer. *Studies in the History of Medieval Science*. Cambridge: Harvard University Press, 1924.

————. "The Abacus and the King's Curia." *EHR* 27(1912):101–6.

————. "Adelard of Bath" *EHR* 26(1911):491–98.

————. "The Reception of Arabic Science in England." *EHR* 30(1915):56–69.

Hawkes, Sonia Chadwick, and Wells, Calvin. "An Anglo-Saxon Obstetric Calamity from Kenworthy, Hampshire." *Medical and Biological Illustration* 25(1975): 47–51.

————. "Crime and Punishment in an Anglo-Saxon Cemetary?" *Antiquity* 49 (1975):118–22.

Herlihy, David. "Life Expectations for Women in Medieval Society." In *The Role of Women in the Middle Ages*, edited by Rosmaris Thee Morewedge, pp. 1–22. Albany: State University of New York Press, 1975.

Herrlinger, Robert. *A History of Medical Illustration From Antiquity to 1700*. Pitman Medical and Scientific Publishing Co., 1970.

Hill, Bennett. *English Cistercian Monasteries and their Patrons in the Twelfth Century*. Urbana and London: University of Illinois Press, 1968.

Hinton, David. *Alfred's Kingdom: Wessex and the South, 800–1500*. London: J. M. Dent and Sons, 1977.

Hodgson, John. *A History of Northumberland*. 7 vols. Newcastle, 1820–58.

Hodgson, Walter E. *The Life of Thomas I, archbishop of York, 1108–1114*. Nottingham, 1909.

Hollister, C. Warren. "Henry I and the Anglo-Norman Magnates." In *Proceedings of the Battle Conference on Anglo-Norman Studies*, edited by R. Allen Brown. pp. 93–107. 2(1979) Woodbridge: Boydell Press, 1980.

_____. "Magnates and Curiales in Early Norman England." *Viator* 7(1977):63–81.

_____. "The Origins of the English Treasury." *EHR* 93(1978):262–75.

Holmes, Richard. "Paulinus of Leeds." *Thoresby Society Publications, Miscellanea* 4 (1895):209–25.

Holmes, Urban T. "The Anglo-Norman Rhymed Chronicle." In *Linguistic and Literary Studies in Honor of Helmut A. Hatzfeld*, edited by Alessandro S. Crisafulli, pp. 231–36. Washington, D.C., 1964.

_____. "Transitions in European Education." In *Twelfth-Century Europe and the Foundations of Modern Society*, edited by Marshall Clagett, Gaines Post, and Robert Reynolds, pp. 15–38.

_____, and Weedon, Frederick R. "Peter of Blois as a Physician." *Speculum* 37 (1962):252–56.

Honeybourne, M. B. "The Leper Houses of the London Area." *Transactions of the London and Middlesex Archaeological Society* 21(1963–67):1–61.

Hughes, Muriel Joy. *Women Healers in Medieval Life and Literature*. 1943. Reprint. New York, 1968.

Hunt, Richard William. "The Disputation of Peter of Cornwall against Symon the Jew." In *Studies in Medieval History Presented to F. M. Powicke*, edited by R. W. Hunt, W. A. Pantin, and R. W. Southern. Oxford: Oxford University Press 1948.

_____, "The Library Abbey of St. Albans." In Parkes and Watson, *Medieval Scribes*, pp. 251–77.

Hurd-Mead, Kate Campbell. "Trotula." *Isis* 14(1930):349–67.

Hurry, Jameison B. *Reading Abbey*. London, 1891.

Jack, R. Ian. "An Archival Case History: The Cartularies and Registers of Llanthony Priory in Gloucestershire." *Journal of the Society of Archivists* 4(1972):370–83.

Jackson, Stanley. "Unusual Mental States in Medieval Europe." *JHM* 37(1972):262–95.

Jadon, Samira. "A Comparison of the Wealth, Prestige, and Medical Works of the Physicians of Salah-al-Din in Egypt and Syria." *BHM* 44(1970):64–75.

_____. "The Physicians of Syria during the Reign of Salah-al-din, 570–589 A.H.. 1174–1193 A.D." *JHM* 25(1970:323–40.

James, Montague Rhodes. *A Descriptive Catalogue of the manuscripts in the Library of Corpus Christi College, Cambridge*. 2 vols. Cambridge, 1912.

_____. *A Descriptive Catalogue of the Manuscripts in the Library of Jesus College, Cambridge*. London, 1895.

_____. "Manuscripts from Essex Monastic Libraries." *Trans. Essex Archaeo. Soc.* n.s. 21(1937):34–46.

Jones, Chester H. "The Chapel of Saint Mary Magdalene at Sturbridge, Cambridge. *Cambridge Antiquarian Society Proceedings* 28(1927):126–50.

Jones, J. G. Penhyn. "Medicine in the Tenth Century: Facts from Welsh Medical Law," *Medicine Illustrated* 5(1951):84–86.

Jones, T. H. "Social Life as Reflected in the Laws of Hywel Dda." In *the Hywel Dda Millenary Volume*, Aberstwyth Studies by members of the University College of Wales, 10(1928).

Kaiser, R. "Laon aux XIe and XIIe siécles." *Revue du Nord* 56(1974):421–26.

Kauffmann, C. M. *Romanesque Manuscripts, 1066–1190*. London: Harvey Miller; New York: New York Graphic Society, 1975.

Kealey, Edward J. *Roger of Salisbury, Viceroy of England* (Berkeley, Los Angeles, and London: University of California Press, 1972.

————. "Anglo-Norman Policy and the Public Welfare." *Albion* 10(1978):341–51.

————. "King Stephen: Government and Anarchy, 1135–1154." *Albion* 6(1974): 201–17.

————. "Recent Writing About Anglo-Norman England." *British Studies Monitor* 9(1979):3–22.

Kemp, Brian R. *Reading Abbey*. Reading, 1968.

————. "The Churches of Berkeley Hernesse." *Trans. Bris. and Glouc. Archaeo. Soc.* 87(1968):96–110.

Ker, Neil Ripley. *Medieval Libraries of Great Britain*. Oxford. Oxford University Press, 1964.

————. *Medieval Manuscripts in British Libraries*. 2 vols. Oxford. Oxford University Press, 1969, 1977.

————. "William of Malmesbury's Handwriting." *EHR* 59(1944):371–76.

————. "The Beginnings of Salisbury Cathedral Library." In *Medieval Learning and Literature: Essays Presented to Richard William Hunt*, edited by J. J. G. Alexander and M. T. Gibson, pp. 23–49. Oxford, 1976.

Kerling, Nellie J. M. "The Foundation of St. Bartholomew's Hospital in West Smithfield, London." *Guildhall Miscellany* 4(1972):137–48.

Kibre, Pearl. "Hippocratic Writings in the Middle Ages." *BHM* 18(1946):371–412.

King, Edmund. *Peterborough Abbey, 1086–1310*. Cambridge: At the University Press, 1973.

————. "The Peterborough *Description Militum* (Henry I)." *EHR* 84(1969):84–101.

Kitson, Peter. "Lapidary Traditions in Anglo-Saxon England: Part I, The Background, the Old English Lapidary." *Anglo-Saxon England* 7(1978):9–60.

Knowles, David. *The Monastic Order in England*. Cambridge. At the University Press, 1940.

————. Brooke, C.N.L.; and London, Vera C. M. *The Heads of Religious Houses: England and Wales, 940–1216* Cambrige: At the University Press, 1972.

————. and Hadcock, R. Neville. *Medieval Religious Houses: England and Wales*. London and New York: St. Martin's Press, 1971.

Könsgen, Ewald. "Zwei unbekannte Briefe zu den Gesta Regum Anglorum des Wilhelm von Malmesbury." *Deutsches Archive für Erforschung des Mittelalters* 31(1975):204–14.

Krappe, Alexander W. "The Historical Background of Philippe de Thaun's *Bestiare*." *Modern Language Notes* 59(1944):325–27.

Kristeller, Paul Oskar. "The School of Salerno." *BHM* 17(1945):138–94.

Lacarra, José M. *Vida de Alfonso el Batallador*. Sargossa, 1971.

Lambrick, Gabrielle. "Abingdon Abbey Administration." *JEH* 17(1966):159–83.

Landon, L. "Everard, bishop of Norwich." *Proceedings of the Suffolk Institute of Archaeology* 20(1930):186–98.

Langston, J. N. "Priors of Llanthony by Gloucester." *Trans. Bris. and Glouc. Archaeo. Soc.* 63(1942):1–143.

Lawn, Brian. *The Salernitan Questions*. Oxford: Oxford University Press, 1963.

Legge, M. Dominica. *Anglo-Norman Literature and Its Background*. Oxford: Oxford University Press, 1963.

_____. "L'influence littéraire de la cour d'Henri Beauclerc," *Mélanges offerts à Rita Lejeune*. Gembloux, 1969. 1:679–87.

Lekai, Louis J. *The Cistercians: Ideals and Reality*. Kent, Ohio: Kent State University Press, 1977.

Lennard, Reginald. *Rural England, 1086–1135*. Oxford: Oxford University Press, 1959.

Le Patourel, John. *The Norman Empire*. Oxford: Oxford University Press, 1976.

Lindberg, David C. *Science in the Middle Ages*. Chicago and London: University of Chicago Press, 1978.

Loewe, Raphael. "Handwashing and the Eyesight in the *Regimen Sanitatis*." *BHM* 30(1956):100–8.

_____. "The Medieval Christian Hebraists of England." *Transactions of the Jewish Historical Society of England* 17(1951–52): 225–50.

Loomis, C. Grant. "Lapidary Medicine," *BHM* 16(1944):319–24.

Lourie, Elena. "The Will of Alfonso I 'El Batallador,' King of Aragon and Navarre: A Reassessment," *Speculum* 50(1975):635–52.

Lowndes, G. Alan. "A History of the Priory of Hatfield Regis, alias Hatfield Broad Oak," *Trans. Essex Archaeo. Soc.* n.s. 2(1884):117–52.

Luscomb, David E. "The Authorship of the *Ysagoge in Theologiam*." *Archives d'Histoire Doctrinale et Littérarie du Moyen Age* 35(1968):7–16.

MacArthur, William. "Medieval Leprosy in the British Isles." *Leprosy Review* 24 (1953):8–19.

McCullough, Florence. *Medieval Latin and French Bestiaries*. Chapel Hill: University of North Carolina Press, 1962.

McGurk, P. "Computus Helperic: Its Transmission in England in the Eleventh and Twelfth Centuries." *Medium Aevum* 43(1974):1–5.

McKeon, Richard. "The Organization of Sciences and the Relation of Cultures in the Twelfth and Thirteenth Centuries." In *The Cultural Context of Medieval Learning*, edited by John Emery Murdoch and Edith Dudley Sylla. Dordrecht and Boston: D. Reidel Co., 1975.

MacKinney, Loren. *Early Medieval Medicine with Special Reference to France and Chartres*. Baltimore: Johns Hopkins University Press, 1937.

_____. *Medical Illustrations in Medieval Manuscripts*. Berkeley and Los Angeles: University of California Press, 1965.

Madox, Thomas. *The History and Antiquities of the Exchequer*. London, 1769.

Majno, Guido. *The Healing Hand: Man and Wound in the Ancient World*. Cambridge: Harvard University Press, 1975.

Mann, Max F. "Der Physiologus des Philipp von Thaün und Seine Quellen." *Anglia* 7(1884):420–68.

Mason, Emma. "Magnates, Curiales, and the Wheel of Fortune." In *Proceedings of the Battle Conference on Anglo-Norman Studies*, edited by R. Allen Brown. pp. 118–40. 2(1979) Woodbridge: Boydell Press, 1980.

Mason, J. F. "The Officers and Clerks of the Norman Earls of Shropshire." *Transactions of the Shropshire Archaeological Society* 56(1957–60):244–57.

Mayr-Harting, Henry. *The Bishops of Chichester, 1075–1207*. Chichester: Chichester City Council, 1963.

_____. "Functions of a Twelfth-Century Recluse." *History* 60(1975);337–52.

Meade, Dorothy M. "The Hospital of Saint Giles at Kepier near Durham, 1112–1545," *Transactions of the Architectural and Archaeological Society of Durham and Northumberland*, n.s. 1(1968):45–58.

Medvei, Victor Cornelius, and Thornton, John L. *The Royal Hospital of Saint Bartholomew, 1123–1973*. London, 1974.

Mercier, Charles. *Leper Hospitals*. London, 1915.

Metlitzki, Dorothee. *The Matter of Araby in Medieval England*. New Haven and London: Yale University Press, 1977.

Meyer, Paul. "Les plus anciens lapidaries français." *Romania* 38(1909):44–70, 254–85, 481–552.

Meyerhof, Max. "Sultan Saladin's Physician on the Transmission of Greek Medicine to the Arabs." *BHM* 18(1945):169–78.

Millás Vallicrosa, José Maria, Nuevos estudios sobre historia de la ciencia espagnõla. Barcelona, 1960.

_____. "La Aportacion Astronomica de Pedro Alfonso." *Sefarad* 3(1943):65–105.

_____. "Un nuevo dato sobre Pedro Alfonso." *Sefarad* 7(1947):136.

Miller, Edward. *The Abbey and Bishopric of Ely*. Cambridge: At the University Press, 1951.

Miller, Timothy. "The Knights of Saint John and the Hospitallers of the Latin West." *Speculum* 53(1978):709–23.

Molland, Einar. "Ut Sapiens Medicus. Medical Vocabulary in St. Benedict's *Regula Monachorum*." *Studia Monastica* 6(1964):173–96.

Moore, Norman. *The History of St. Bartholomew's Hospital*. London, 1918.

_____. *The Physician in English History*. Cambridge: At the University Press, 1913.

Morson, John. "The English Cistercians and the Bestiary," *Bulletin of the John Rylands Library* 39(1956–57):146–70.

Mundy, John H. "Hospitals and Leprosaries in Twelfth- and Thirteenth-Century Toulouse." In *Essays on Medieval Life and Thought Presented in Honor of Austin P. Evans*, edited by J. H. Mundy and R. W. Emery. New York: Columbia University Press, 1955.

Mynors, Roger A. B. *Durham Cathedral Manuscripts*. Oxford: At the University Press, 1939.

Nash-Williams, V. E. *The Early Christian Monuments of Wales*. Cardiff, 1950.

Nelson, Lynn H. "Rotrou of Perche and the Aragonese Reconquest." *Traditio* 26(1970):113–33.

Newton, Robert R. *Medieval Chronicles of the Rotation of the Earth*. Baltimore: Johns Hopkins University Press, 1972.

Nicholson, Joseph, and Burn, Richard. *History and Antiquities of Cumberland and Westmorland*. London, 1777.

O'Callaghan, Joseph. *A History of Medieval Spain*. Ithaca: Cornell University Press, 1975.

Oliver, George. *History of Exeter*. Exeter, 1861.

O'Malley, Austin P., F.S.C., "Petrus Alfonsi," *New Catholic Encyclopedia*. 11:209. Washington, D.C., 1967.

Orme, Nicholas. *English Schools in the Middle Ages*. London: Methuen, 1973.

Owen, Dorothy. *Church and Society in Medieval Lincolnshire*. Lincoln, 1971.

Pagel-Koll, Magda. "The Surgery of Jamerius." *BHM* 28(1954):471–88.

Palgrave, Francis. *Collected Historical Works*. 7 vols. Cambridge: At the University Press, 1921.

Parkes, M. B., and Watson, Andrew, eds. *Medieval Scribes, Manuscripts, and Libraries: Essays Presented to N. R. Ker*. London: Scolar Press, 1978.

Partner, Nancy F., *Serious Entertainments: The Writing of History in Twelfth-Century England*. Chicago and London: University of Chicago Press, 1977.

Parton, J. *History of the Hospital and Parish of St. Giles in the Fields*. London, 1822.

Pinto, Lucille B. "Medical Science and Superstition: A Report on a Unique Medical Scroll of the Eleventh-Twelfth Century." *Manuscripta* 17(1973):12–21.

Piper, A. J. "The Libraries of the Monks of Durham." In Parkes and Watson, *Medieval Scribes*. pp. 213–49.

Platt, Colin. *The Medieval Town*. New York: David McKay Co., 1976.

Poulle, Emmanuel. "Les Instruments astronomiques de l'Occident latin aux XIᵉ et XIIᵉ siècles." *Cahiers de Civilisation Médiévale* 15(1972):27–40.

Powell, W. R., "The Essex Fees of the Honor of Richmond." *Trans. Essex Archaeo. Soc.*, 3d ser. 1(1964):179–89.

Reece, Richard. "The Knights Hospitaller at Quenington." *Trans. Bris. and Glouc. Archaeo. Soc.* 93(1974):131–35.

Richards, Peter. *The Medieval Leper and His Northern Heirs*. London: Rowman and Littlefield, 1977.

Richardson, Henry Gerald. *The English Jewry under the Angevin Kings*. London, 1960.

Riddle, John M. "Dioscorides." *Dictionary of Scientific Biography* 4(1971):119–23.

————. "Lithotherapy in the Middle Ages: Lapidaries Considered as Medical Texts." *Pharmacy in History* 12(1970):39–50.

————. "Theory and Practice in Medieval Medicine." *Viator* 5(1974):157–84.

Ritchie, R. L. Graeme. *The Normans in Scotland*. Edinburgh, 1954.

————. "The Date of the *Voyage of St. Brendan*." *Medium Aevum* 19(1950): 64–66.

Robbins, Rossell Hope, "Medical Manuscripts in Middle English." *Speculum* 44(1970):393–415.

Roberts, George. "Llanthony Priory, Monmouthshire." *Archaeologia Cambrensis* 1(1841):202–43.

Roberts, R. S. "Epidemics and Social History." *Medical History* 12(1968):305–16.

Robinson, J. Armitage. *Gilbert Crispin, abbot of Westminster* Cambridge: At the University Press, 1911.

Rohde, Eleanour. *The Old English Herbals*. London, 1922.

Rose-Troup, Frances. *Exeter Vignettes*. Manchester: History of Exeter Research Group, 1942.

Roth, Cecil. *A History of the Jews in England*. Oxford: Oxford University Press, 1949.

Round, John Horace. *The Commune of London*. Westminster, 1899.

_____. *Feudal England*. London, 1895.

_____. "Bernard, the King's Scribe." *EHR* 14(1899):417–30.

_____. "The Earliest Essex Medical Man." *Trans. Essex Archaeo. Soc.*, n.s. 12(1913):337–38.

_____. "The Origins of St. Botolph's Priory, Colchester." *Trans. Essex Archaeo. Soc.*, n.s. 3(1889):267–72.

Rubin, Stanley. *Medieval English Medicine*. London and Newton Abbot: David and Charles, 1974.

Sabin, Arthur. "St. Augustine's Abbey and the Berkeley Churches." *Trans. Bris. and Glouc. Archaeo. Soc.* 89(1970):90–98.

Saffron, Morris Harold. *Maurus of Salerno, Twelfth-Century Optimus Physicus*. Philadelphia: American Philosophical Society, 1972.

Salter, Herbert E. "The City of Oxford in the Middle Ages." *EHR* 14(1929):97–105.

Saltman, Avrom. *Theobald, Archbishop of Canterbury*. London, 1956.

Sanford, Eva Matthews. "Honorius, Presbyter and Scholasticus." *Speculum* 23(1948): 397–425.

Sarton, George. *Introduction to the History of Science*. 3 vols. Baltimore, 1927–48.

Saunders, H. W. "A History of Coxford Priory." *Norfolk Archaeology* 17(1910): 284–370.

Sawyer, Peter. *From Roman Britain to Norman England*. New York and London: St. Martin's Press, 1978.

Scammell, G. V. *Hugh du Puiset, bishop of Durham*. Cambridge: At the University Press, 1956.

Schwarzbaum, Haim. "International Folklore Motifs in Pedro Alphonsi's *Disciplina Clericalis*." *Sefarad* 21(1961):267–99, 22(1962):17–59, 321–44, 23(1963):54–73.

Scullard, H. H. *Roman Britain: Outpost of the Empire*. London: Thames and Hudson, 1979.

Searle, Eleanor. *Lordship and Community: Battle Abbey and its Banlieu, 1066–1538* Toronto: Pontifical Institute of Medieval Studies, 1974.

_____. "Battle Abbey and Exemption: The Forged Charters." *EHR* 83(1968): 449–80.

Seide, Jacob. "Medicine and Natural History in the Itinerary of Rabbi Benjamin of Tudela (1100–1177)." *BHM* 28(1954):401–7.

Shields, Hugh. "Philippe de Thaon, auteur de *Livre de Sibylle?*" *Romania* 85(1964): 455–77.

Sigerist, Henry. "Early Medieval Medical Texts in Manuscripts in Vendôme," *BHM* 14(1943):68–113.

_____. "The Latin Medical Literature of the Early Middle Ages." *JHM* 13(1958): 127–46.

————. "Materia Medica in the Middle Ages." *BHM* 7(1939):417–23.

————. "A Salernitan Student's Surgical Notebook." *BHM* 14(1943):505–16.

Simanis, Joseph G. *National Health Systems in Eight Countries.* Washington: U.S. Department of Health, Education, and Welfare, 1975.

Singer, Charles. "A Review of the Medical Literature of the Dark Ages with a Text of about 1110." *Proceedings of the Royal Society of Medicine* 10(1916–17):105–60.

————. "A Legend of Salerno: How Constantine the African Brought the Art of Medicine to the Christians." *Johns Hopkins Hospital Bulletin* 28(1917): 64–69.

————. "Early English Magic and Medicine." *Proceedings of the British Academy* 18(1919–20):341–74.

————. "The Herbal in antiquity and its Transmission to Later Ages." *Journal of Hellenic Studies* 47(1927):1–52.

Singer, Dorothea Waley. "Survey of Medical Manuscripts in the British Isles dating before the Sixteenth Century." *Proceedings of the Royal Society of Medicine* 12(1918–19):96–107.

Slade, C. F. "Excavations at Reading Abbey, 1964–1967." *Berkshire Archaeological Journal* 66(1971–72):65–116.

Smalley, Beryl. *The Becket Conflict and the Schools.* Oxford: Oxford University Press, 1973.

————. "Master Ivo of Chartres." *EHR* 50(1935):680–86.

————. "Gilbertus Universalis, bishop of London (1128–1134) and the Problem of the Glossa Ordinaria," *Recherches de théologie ancienne et médiévale* 7(1935): 235–62.

————. "Ralph of Flaix on Leviticus." *Recherches de théologie ancienne et médiévale* 35(1968):35–82.

Smith, R.A.L. "John of Tours, bishop of Bath, 1088–1122." *Downside Review* 60(1942):132–41.

Southern, Richard W. *Saint Anslem and His Biographer.* Cambridge: At the University Press, 1963.

————. *Medieval Humanism.* New York: Harper and Row, Harper Torchbacks, 1970.

Stenton, Doris Mary. *The English Woman in History.* London and New York, 1957.

Stenton, Frank Merry. "St. Benet of Holme and the Norman Conquest." *EHR* 37(1922):225–35.

Stiefel, Tina. "Science, Reason, and Faith in the Twelfth Century: The Cosmologists' Attack on Tradition." *Journal of European History* 6(1976):1–16.

————. "The Heresy of Science: A Twelfth-Century Conceptual Revolution." *Isis* 68(1977):347–62.

Stubbs, William. *The Foundation of Waltham Abbey.* Oxford: Oxford University Press, 1861.

Studer, Paul, and Evans, Joan. *Anglo-Norman Lapidaries.* Paris, 1924.

Sudhoff, Karl. "Tabellen, Bild und Merkschemata zur Kauterienanwendung bei Erkrankungen." In *Beitrage zur Geschichte der Chirurgie im Mittelalter.* Leipzig, 1914. 1:75–124.

Sumption, Jonathan. *Pilgrimage: An Image of Medieval Religion.* London: Faber and Faber, 1975.

Talbot, Charles H. *Medicine in Medieval England.* London, 1967.

_____. "A Letter from Bartholomew of Salerno to King Louis of France." *BHM* 30(1956):321–28.

_____. "A Letter of Roger Abbot of Byland." *Analecta Sacri Ordinis Cisterciensis* 7(1951):218–31.

_____. "A Medieval Physician's Vade Mecum." *JHM* 16(1961):213–33.

_____. "Some Notes on Anglo-Saxon Medicine." *Medical History* 9(1965):156–69.

_____, and Hammond, Eugene A., *The Medical Practitioners in Medieval England: A Biographical Register*. London: Wellcome Historical Medical Library, 1965.

Thompson, John D., and Goldin, Grace. *The Hospital: A Social and Architectural History*. New Haven: Yale University Press, 1978.

Thomson, Rodney M. " 'Liber Marii de Elementis,' the Work of a Hitherto Unknown Salernitan Master." *Viator* 3(1972):179–89.

_____. "The Library of Bury St. Edmunds Abbey in the Eleventh and Twelfth Centuries." *Speculum* 47(1972):617–45.

_____. The Reading of William of Malmesbury," *Revue Bénédictine* 85(1975): 362–402.

_____. "The Reading of William of Malmesbury: Addenda et Corrigenda." *Revue Bénédictine* 86(1976):327–35.

_____. "The Reading of William of Malmesbury: Further Additions and Reflections." *Revue Bénédictine* 89(1979):313–24.

_____. "The 'Scriptorium' of William of Malmesbury." In Parkes and Watson, *Medieval Scribes*. pp. 117–142.

_____. "A Twelfth-Century Letter from Bury St. Edmunds." *Revue Bénédictine* 82(1972):87–97.

_____. "Two Twelfth-Century Poems on the Regnum Sacerdotium Problem in England." *Revue Bénédictine* 83(1973):312–25.

_____. "Two Versions of a Saint's Life from St. Edmund's Abbey." *Revue Bénédictine* 84(1974):383–408.

_____. "William of Malmesbury as Historian and Man of Letters." *JEM* 29(1978): 387–413.

_____. "William of Malmesbury and the Letters of Alcuin." *Medievalia et Humanistica*, n.s. 8(1977):147–61.

_____. "William of Malmesbury and Some Other Western Writers on Islam." *Medievalia et Humanistica*. n.s. 6(1975):179–88.

Thorndike, Lynn. *A History of Magic and Experimental Science*. 8 vols. New York, 1923–58.

_____. "Of the Cylinder Called the Horloge of Travellers." *Isis* 13(1929–30): 51–52.

_____. "John of Seville." *Speculum* 34(1959):20–38.

_____. "The True Place of Astrology in the History of Science." *Isis* 46(1955): 273–78.

_____, and Kibre, Pearl. *A Catalogue of Incipits of Medieval Scientific Writings in Latin*. Cambridge, Mass.: Medieval Academy of America, 1963.

Turner, Cuthbert, H. "The Earliest List of Durham Manuscripts." *Journal of Theological Studies* 19(1918):121–32.

Turner, Ralph V. "The Miles Literatus in Twelfth- and Thirteenth-Century England: How Rare a Phenomenon?" *AHR* 83(1978):928–45.

Tuttle, Edward F. "The Trotula and Old Dame Trot: A Note on the Lady of Salerno." *BHM* 50(1976):61–72.

Urry, William J. *Canterbury Under the Angevin Kings*. London: Athlone, 1967.

Vaughn, Sally M. "Saint Anselm: Reluctant Archbishop." *Albion* 6(1974): 242–45.

Vercauteren, F. "Les Médicins dans les principautés de la Belgique et du Nord de la France, du VIII^c au XIII^c siècle." *LeMoyen Age* 57(1951):61–92.

Voights, Linda Ersham. "A New Look at a Manuscript Containing the Old English Translation of the *Hebrarium Apulei*." *Manuscripta* 20(1976):40–61.

Watkin, Hugh R. *History of Totnes Priory and Its Medieval Town*. 2 vols. Torquay, 1914–17.

Watson, John. *Memoirs of the Earls of Warren and Surrey*. 2 vols. Warrington, 1782.

Wells, Calvin. *Bones, Bodies, and Disease*. New York: Praeger, 1964.

————. "A Leper Cemetary at South Acre, Norfolk." *Medieval Archaeology* 11(1967):242–48.

White, Lynn, Jr., "Natural Science and Naturalistic Art in the Middle Ages." *AHR* 52(1947):421–35.

————. "Eilmer of Malmesbury: An Eleventh-Century Aviator." *Technology and Culture* 2(1961):97–111.

————. "The Study of Medieval Technology, 1924–1974: Personal Reflections." *Technology and Culture* 16(1975):519–30.

White, T. H. *The Book of Beasts*. London, 1954.

Wickersheimer, Ernest. *Dictionnaire biographique des médecins en France au moyen age*. 2 vols. Paris, 1936.

Wightman, W. E. *The Lacy Family in England and Normandy, 1066–1194*. Oxford: Oxford University Press, 1966.

Williams, Arthur Lukyn. *Adversus Judaeos*. Cambridge: At the University Press, 1935.

Williams, L. F. Rushbrook. "William the Chamberlain and Luton Church." *EHR* 28(1913):719–30.

Williams. T. W. "Gloucestershire Medieval Libraries." *Trans. Bris. and Glouc. Archaeo. Soc.* 31(1908):76–177.

Woodings, Ann F. "The Medical Resources and Practice of the Crusader States in Syria and Palestine, 1093–1193." *Medical History* 25(1971):268–77.

Woolley, Reginald Maxwell. *Catalogue of the Manuscripts of Lincoln Cathedral Library*. Oxford: Oxford University Press, 1927.

Wright, John Kirkland. *The Geographical Lore of the Time of the Crusades*. New York, 1925.

————. "Notes on the Knowledge of Latitudes and Longitudes in the Middle Ages." *Isis* 5(1923):75–98.

Yeldman, Florence A. "Fraction Tables of Hermanus Contractus." *Speculum* 3(1928):240–45.

NOTES

CHAPTER I

1. Evidence for the physicians is discussed in Chapters 2, 3 and Appendix 1. The hospital foundations are documented in Chapter 4 and Appendix 2.

2. Bonser, *Medical Background*, pp. 58, 92; see also his "Epidemics During the Anglo-Saxon Period," and Creighton, *History of Epidemics in Britain*, 1:15–16, 29–31. Note the criticism of Creighton by Roberts, "Epidemics and Social History."

3. William of Malmesbury, *G.P.*, 2:335–37; Orderic Vitalis, 4:79–81. The physicians present included Bishop Gilbert Maminot of Lisieux, Abbot Gontard of Jumièges, and several others, perhaps John of Tours and Abbot Baldwin of Bury. Moore, *Physician in English History*, pp. 10–2, suggests that the Conqueror suffered an obstruction of the large intestine.

4. Much of the evidence comes from annual entries in the *Anglo-Saxon Chronicle*; see also n. 2 above. It may not have been accidental that the year 1112 also witnessed a dramatic revival of the cult of the Saxon pseudo-saint, Earl Waltheof, who rebelled against the Conquest and became a political victim of the Conqueror's wrath; see Orderic Vitalis, 3:349–51.

5. The most useful general works are Talbot, *Medicine in Medieval England*, and Rubin, *Medieval English Medicine*. One of the best reviews of learning and medicine can be found in Barlow, *The English Church*, pp. 217–67.

6. Talbot, "Anglo-Saxon Medicine."

7. For example, in 1119 Archbishop Thurstan of York remained in Paris to be bled; Hugh the Chanter, *Church of York*, p. 70.

8. For occulists in Roman Britain see Scullard, *Roman Britain*, pp. 144–45.

9. For other discussions see Gransden, "Realistic Observation," and Stiefel, "Science, Reason and Faith."

10. Singer, "Survey of Medical Manuscripts"; Beddie, "Libraries in the Twelfth Century," p. 8; Robbins, "Medical Manuscripts," p. 393. English language versions pick up again as early as the thirteenth century.

11. Large sections of this work, now Saint John's College, Oxford, Ms. 17, are printed, illustrated, and analyzed by Singer, "Medical Literature of the Dark Ages," and by Southern, *Medieval Humanism*, plates 3, 6, 7, 8. Southern's stimulating essays contain many valuable insights into twelfth-century marvels and sciences.

12. Apuleius Barbarus: this is Oxford University, Bodleian Library, Ms. 130. See also Voights, "The Old English Translation of the *Herbrarium Apulei*"; Rubin, *Medieval English Medicine*, pp. 45–47; Rohde, *Old English Herbals*; Thomson, "The Library of Bury Saint Edmunds."

13. A similar collection of medical books (B.L., Ms. Harley 1585) even contained an invocation to Mother Earth. This manuscript was formerly considered a late eleventh- early twelfth-century English work; Singer, "Magic and Medicine," pp. 372–73; Bonser, *Medical Background*, pp. 431–32; MacKinney, *Medical Illustrations*, pp. 137–38. Recent research, however, indicates that it comes from the Mosan area of France about 1175; Kauffman, *Romanesque Manuscripts*, p. 126.

15. For a brilliant introduction see James, ed. *The Bestiary*. The particular copy edited here is Cambridge University Library, Ms. Ii, 4. 26, an exceptionally fine twelfth-century work. For a translation see White, *Book of Beasts*. The Cambridge bestiary may be from the Cistercian abbey of Revesby, in Lincolnshire; Morson, "English Cistercians and the Bestiary," p. 167. Two men called medicus were associated with Revesby—William was there in 1142 and Ailred was abbot from 1142 to 1147. Ailred frequently quoted from the bestiary in his many writings. Cronin, in "The Bestiary and the Medieval Mind," has argued that these works exhibit an interest in natural fact, as did Forbes, "Medical Lore in the Bestiaries." See also McCullough, *Medieval Latin and French Bestiaries*. For guides to the use of minerals in medicine see Riddle, "Lithotherapy," and Evans and Serjeantson, eds., *English Medieval Lapidaries*, p. xi.

16. Druce, "The Caladrius and Its Legend," and "Medieval Bestiaries and their Influence." For examples of the caladrius in bestiaries and medical books, see White, *Book of Beasts*, p. 115, and MacKinney, *Medical Illustrations*, pp. 22, 52, 113, 114, and plates 16, and 49. Authors such as Philip of Thaon, Honorius of Autun, Ailred of Rievaulx, and Hugh of Saint Victor mention the caladrius.

17. For one collection, the *Peri-Didaxeon* (*Medical Doctrines*), copied about 1150, see Cockayne, ed., *Leechdoms, Wortcunning, and Starcraft*, 3:83–145.

18. For examples see MacKinney, *Medical Illustrations*, pp. 52, 69, 114, 137, 143, 160, plate 49.

19. For one of the best accounts of the value of early techniques, see Riddle, "Theory and Practice in Medieval Medicine," esp. p. 169.

20. Southern, *Medieval Humanism*, pp. 164–65.

21. Chroniclers like Reginald of Durham and William of Newburgh were also very interested in medicine. For John of Worcester see Flint, "The Chronicle of 'Florence.'" For Henry of Huntingdon see Partner, *Serious Entertainments*, pp. 11–50.

22. White, "Eilmer of Malmesbury." For Saewulf see Wright, *Travels in Palestine*, pp. 31–50; William of Malmesbury, *G.P.*, p. 282. Robert de Veneys, physician of Henry II, was a monk of Malmesbury and abbot there 1171/2–1180. Presumably he arrived there late in William's life; see *H.R.H.*, p. 55.

23. The literature on Malmesbury is voluminous, but the best places to begin are Farmer, "William of Malmesbury's Life and Works," and Thomson, "The Reading of William of Malmesbury," and "The Reading of William of Malmesbury: Addenda et Corrigenda." See also Thomson's "William of Malmesbury and Other Writers," and "William of Malmesbury as Historian."

24. William of Malmesbury, *G.R.*, 1:103.

25. Malmesbury had evidently seen an Arabic treatise on embryology; Thomson, "The Reading of William of Malmesbury," p. 383. He also knew works on Islamic computation and general theology.

26. For example, his *Life of St. Wulstan*, pp. 41, 52. William even reports that Gregory, the Malmesbury physician, could not cure all his patients, and men like Ernulf de Hesdin, an important baron of Henry I, had to turn to Saint Aldhelm for relief; William of Malmesbury, *G.P.*, p. 437.

27. Robert of Hereford's writings were well known to both William of Malmesbury and John of Worcester. One of the three surviving copies of Hereford's work on the calendar was made by William, who also knew Walcher's studies.

28. The availability of pills has been unnecessarily questioned; see contemporary references to them in Talbot, trans., *Christina of Marykate*, pp. 123, 125; Fulbert of Chartres, pp. 47–48, referring to laxatives; Peter the Venerable 2:383; Talbot, "A Letter from Bartholomew of Sa-

lerno." None of the above material suggests that people were popping pills in the twelfth century. For the possibility of anesthesia, see Rubin, *Medieval English Medicine*, p. 137, citing the biography of Saint Kentigern (d. 612) by Bishop John of Glasgow (1175–99), edited by Forbes, *Historians of Scotland*, 5:35. The bishop referred to a potion, evidently in common use in his own time, which enabled a patient to be oblivious to pain endured in surgery or cauterization. MacKinney, *Medical Illustrations*, pp. 53–54, reproduces an eleventh-century miniature which may show a physician offering a patient a sporific sponge before surgery.

29. Downer, ed. and trans., *Leges Henrici Primi*, pp. 245, 271; see also Bonser's chapter, "Mental Disease and Devil Possession," in his *Medical Background*, pp. 257–63. Orderic Vitalis (4:275) records an interesting, possibly fictitious, case of a man in Norway who insanely murdered a priest at Mass. For punishment he lost his hands and feet and was blinded. Then, fitted with iron fingers, he was taken into the household of David of Scotland where the man repaid the charity by killing the earl's infant son. He was consequently condemned to be bound to four wild horses and torn apart.

Heavenly vengeance was sometimes thought to cause disease. For example, a stroke suffered by Bishop Richard de Beaumais of London was said to be brought on by Saint Osith's (d. c. 700) anger at the lord's alienating some lands of her shrine. When he recovered he built a monastery of Austin canons in her honor at Chich. For the more common belief in purely natural causation for disease, see Finucane, *Miracles and Pilgrims*, pp. 72–75.

30. Geoffrey of Monmouth, *Kings of Britain*, p. 196.

31. Hinton, *Alfred's Kingdom*, pp. 119, 145. 191; Barlow, ed., *Winton Domesday*, p. 284.

32. Until the study appears that C. Warren Hollister is preparing for the University of California Press, one had best begin with Southern's perceptive essay, "King Henry I," first delivered in 1962 and revised for his *Medieval Humanism*, pp. 206–33. Hollister's most recent statement is contained in a joint article with Baldwin, "The Rise of Administrative Kingship." King Stephen has received more attention; see David, *King Stephen*; Cronne, *The Reign of King Stephen*; Appleby, *The Troubled Reign of King Stephen*.

33. Kealey, *Roger of Salisbury*, esp. pp. 26–81.

34. Kealey, "Anglo-Norman Policy."

35. For Matilda's status, see Southern, *Saint Anselm*, pp. 183–93.

36. William of Malmesbury, *G.R.*, 2:494; *Abingdon Chronicle*, 2:50.

37. Kealey, *Roger of Salisbury*, pp. 31, 40–41; the anonymous author of the *Leges Henrici* praised Matilda in his prologue.

38. William of Malmesbury, *G.R.*, 2:494; Ritchie, *Normans in Scotland*, p. 126. Adelard of Bath evidently also sang for Matilda. For the recent discovery that Matilda commissioned Malmesbury's major work, see Thomson, "William of Malmesbury as Historian," p. 391; Ewald Könsgen, "Zwei unbekannte Briefe."

39. Ritchie, "Date of the *Voyage of St. Brendan*"; Legge, *Anglo-Norman Literature*. The same church door on which the caladrius was carved also exhibits a ship atop a whale's back; Benedict, pp. cxxi. 22.

40. William of Malmesbury, *G.R.*, 2:494; *Aldgate Cartulary*, pp. 223–24; *Regesta*, 2, nos. 525, 526, 897, 902, 908, 909, 1090, 1108, 1186.

41. Baker, *Medieval London*, p. 41; It was rents from this wharf that endowed Saint Giles Hospital; Honeybourne, "Leper Houses." For the bridges, see *V.C.H., Essex*, 2:116.

42. Honeybourne, "Leper Houses," p. 5, citing the chronicler Robert of Gloucester. For the reputed miracles see Barlow, *Edward the Confessor*, p. 270.

43. Philip's ecclesiastical calendar was sent to his uncle Humphrey, who was a chaplain of Eudo Dapifer (d. 1120), a well-known court figure and hospital patron. In old age the canon wrote a work on the Sibylline books for Empress Matilda. For a translation of his bestiary, computus, and lapidary, see Wright, *Popular Treatises on Science*. See also Krappe, Philippe de Thäun's *Bestiaire*"; McCullough, *Medieval Latin and French Bestiaries*, pp. 47–54; Mann, "Der Physiologus"; Shields, "Philippe de Thaon." For Adeliza's literary interests, see Holmes, "Anglo-Norman Rhymed Chronicle"; Legge, *Anglo-Norman Literature*, pp. 8–26, and "L'influence litteraire."

44. William of Malmesbury, *G.R.*, 2:485. For the elephant see Ritchie, *Normans in Scotland*, p. 120. The reports of green men and valuable cups are from William of Newburgh *Historia Rerum Anglicarum*, p. 85; see also Partner, *Serious Entertainments*, p. 122.

45. Ritchie, *Normans in Scotland*, p. 112, citing Turgot's life of Margaret.

46. Barlow, *Edward the Confessor*, pp. 247–49, 273; B.L. Ms. Sloane 475, cited in Thorndike, *History of Magic*, 1:725–26.

47. The classic study is Bloch, *Les rois thaumaturges*, which was recently translated by Anderson as *The Royal Touch*. This analysis must now be substantially revised in the light of Barlow's significant critique, "The King's Evil." See also Bonser, *Medical Background*, pp. 270–76; Barlow, *Edward the Confessor*, pp. 256–85.

48. William of Malmesbury, *Vita Wulfstani*, pp. 30, 57. For Goscelin's *Vita S. Edithe*, see Barlow, *Edward the Confessor*, p. 271; Douglas, *William the Conqueror*, pp. 254–55. For Milburga see William of Malmesbury, *G.R.*, 2:222.

49. Douglas, *William the Conqueror*, p. 254; Professor Barlow would not accept this view.

50. William of Malmesbury, *G.R.*, 1:273; Barlow, *Edward the Confessor*, pp. 270–73. The translation is from Barlow, "The King's Evil," p. 17. Malmesbury seems to be responding to a charge by Guibert of Nogent that English kings could not cure disorders. In describing the woman's condition, William related that the humors had abundantly collected about her neck.

51. Among those believing that Henry did practice miraculous healing are Gerould, "King Arthur and Politics," p. 43; David C. Douglas, *The Norman Fate* (Berkeley and Los Angeles: University of California Press, 1976), p. 89. For Henry's theory, see Ritchie, *Normans in Scotland*, pp. 101, 112; Christopher Brooke, *The Saxon and the Norman Kings* (London, 1963), pp. 195–96. Barlow, "The King's Evil," p. 26, finds it incredible that Henry I could have "touched," at least for scrofula.

52. Talbot, *Medicine in Medieval England*, p. 55.

53. For a fine review see Amundsen, "Medieval Canon Law." Bonser, *Medical Background*, p. 172, pointed out that as early as 877 a provincial synod at Ratisbon forbade eccleciastics to study medicine. For the decrees of the First Lateran Council see Flint, "Works of Honorius Augustodunensis." Knowles, *Monastic Order in England*, p. 518, believed that these regulations were not operative in England.

54. William of Malmesbury, *Vita Wulfstani*, pp. 27–28.

55. Smalley, "Ralph of Flaix," p. 37.

CHAPTER II

1. Downer, ed. and trans. *Leges Henrici Primi*, p. 299. For similar references in Saxon laws and penitentials see Bonser, *Medical Background*, pp. 105–08.

2. These identifications were made by the late Calvin Wells, a former practicing surgeon and leading authority on medieval medicine. For a brief summary of his work, see Brown, *Anglo-Saxon England*, pp. 98–100. Not all medical cases were so successful; see Hawkes and Wells, "An Anglo-Saxon Obstetric Calamity."

3. Finucane, *Miracles and Pilgrims*, p. 59; Bethell, "Miracles of St. Ithamar." Another catalog of miracle stories included an account of a woman who had consulted many physicians on several occasions. Kemp, trans., "Miracles of St. James." Many similar references could be added.

4. For a valuable introduction to the techniques and benefits of medieval prosopography, see George Beech, "Prosopography," in *Medieval Studies: An Introduction*, ed. James Powell (Syracuse: Syracuse University Press, 1976) pp. 151–84.

5. Eadmer, *Life of St. Anselm*, p. 63. For Hugh's illness see Vaughn, "Saint Anselm." The Rule of Saint Benedict said twice that an abbot should act as a wise physician; see Molland, "Ut Sapiens Medicus." For an analysis of the popular religious use of some medical terminology, see Arbesmann, "Concept of 'Christus Medicus.' "

6. An example of leech as a patronymic can be found in a grant of William de Friville that was witnessed by Martin le Leche, William le Leche, and Roger le Leche, among others; P.R.O., Ms. Ancient Deeds, A 12132. For terms such as *physicus* and *cirurgicus*, see Bullough, *Medicine as a Profession*; MacKinney, *Early Medieval Medicine*, pp. 142–45. The word *apothecarius* was used, and *obstetrix* was even applied to a wise woman in the early twelfth century, according to Vercauteren, "Les Médecins," p. 66.

7. *Historical Manuscripts Commission, Ninth Report*, p. 62. Two barbers (*rasori*), Baldwin and William, appear in Oxford in 1129–30; *31 Henry I*, pp. 3, 6. Baldwin was responsible for

the large sum of ten pounds, but there is no indication either had any medical or barber-surgeon responsibilities.

8. Ibid.

9. Miller, *Abbey and Bishopric of Ely*, p. 283.

10. Orderic Vitalis, 2:77; Hurd-Mead, "Trotula"; Tuttle, "Old Dame Trot"; Engbring, "Saint Hildegard." About 1136 Heludis medica, evidently a laywoman, practiced in France; Wickersheimer, *Dictionnaire Biographique*, 1:273. Euphemia, abbess of Wherwell, was an active physician. Hughes, *Women Healers*, p. 117, dated her career 1126–1157, but actually she died in 1257; *H.R.H.*, p. 222.

11. Herlihy, "Life Expectations for Women."

12. For Bartholomew see Farmer, *Oxford Dictionary of Saints*, p. 30. For Siward, see Bethell, "Richard of Belemis," p. 305. For Norman see Round, "St. Botolph's Priory." For Baldwin see Davis, "Monks of St. Edmunds," p. 236. For additional instances of Saxons hidden within the records see Sawyer, *From Roman Britain to Norman England*, pp. 255–59.

13. Jones, "Welsh Medical Law," pp. 84–86, has demonstrated what important details can be wrung from limited early sources. See also Richard, trans., *The Laws of Hywel Dda*, esp. pp. 24, 41, 63; Jones, "Social Life as Reflected in the Laws of Hywel Dda"; Cowley, *Monastic Order in South Wales*, p. 4; Cule, "Court Mediciner." Physicians frequently play a role in Irish sagas and legends, and sometimes their personal names are given.

14. John of Salisbury, *Metalogicon*, pp. 17–19. See also Clanchy, "Moderni in Education"; Smalley, *Becket Conflict*, p. 87.

15. Gunther, *Early Science in Oxford*, p. 2. The chronicle source for Cambridge, the so-called pseudo-Ingulf of Crowland, *P.L.* 175:lxxv, has little merit. Orderic Vitalis mentioned no such creation, even though he visited Crowland several times. Nor, despite considerable biographical detail, does Orderic ever call Geoffrey a physician. On the other hand, considering Saint Evroult's strong medical tradition, Geoffrey could easily have received training there. The frequently inaccurate Dubreuil-Chambardel, *Les Médecins*, p. 165, accepted this, but so did the reliable Hammond, "Physicians in Medieval English Religious Houses," p. 109, and Holmes, "Transitions in European Education," p. 22 (wrongly attributing the account to Orderic Vitalis). Geoffrey was not listed as a physician by Talbot and Hammond, *Medical Practitioners*, nor by me.

16. Barrow, ed., *Regesta Regum Scottorum*, 1:167, no. 69 (a grant of King David, 1124x1140). Arnold and Ralph, masons at Crowland and Saint Paul's, were evidently called master as certainly was Master Hugh, the famous artist at Bury Saint Edmunds; see Harvey, *English Medieval Architects*.

17. Thurgis the doctor (Gurgici doctoris) attested for Earl Ranulf of Chester in 1121x1129; *Chester Cartulary*, p. 50. Walcher, the famed scientist and prior of Malvern, was described as Doctor Walcherus on his tombstone; Dugdale, *Monasticon*, 3:442. Master Hamo, the chancellor of Lincoln Cathedral, appeared as Hamo doctor about 1150; Stenton, ed., *Danelaw*, no. 283; Greenway, ed., *Le Neve's "Fasti,"* 3:16, 156. At Fontevrault in 1154 a Matheo doctore ducis witnessed a charter of Duke Henry; *Regesta*, 3, no. 331. This sounds more medical than academic. Married priests at Hexham, men who were ancestors of Ailred of Rievaulx, were often called by the honorable title of *laerow* (doctor).

18. Scammell, *Hugh du Puiset*, p. 10, no. 3. Paulinus of Leeds is an interesting fellow in his own right, but he has sometimes been confused with Paulinus, the physician of York. For a thorough study of celibacy, see Brooke, "Gregorian Reform in Action."

19. Craster, "Miracles of Farne," p. 103, and "Miracles of St. Cuthbert."

20. Orderic Vitalis, who considered himself quite a stylist, described Gilbert Maminot as a medicus and as an archiater, 5:8, 11. He used the latter term several other times, e.g., 1:89, 4:176, 317, 5:19.

21. William of Malmesbury, *G.P.*, p. 145.

22. Roger of Howden, 1:168–69; William of Newburgh, *Historia Rerum Anglicarum*, pp. 28–29. The contemporary historians Symeon of Durham and Hugh the Chanter do not record this tale. See also Partner, *Serious Entertainments*, pp. 69–73.

23. William of Malmesbury, *G.R.*, 2:479; Vercauteren, "Les Médecins," pp. 61–92. An earlier charter of Baldwin had been attested by a Walter medicus, presumably one of his own retainers.

24. See also Thomas on Monmouth, *St. William of Norwich*, p. 209.

25. Talbot, ed. and trans., *Christina of Marykate*, p. 123; Daniel, *Ailred of Rievaulx*, pp. 34, 49.

26. Jane Tibbets Schulenberg, "Sexism and the Celestial Gynaeceum from 500 to 1210," *Journal of Medieval History* 4(1978):129. 42 percent of all male saints lived past 70 and another 24 percent died between 61 and 70.

27. Botfield, ed., *Catalogues of Durham Cathedral*, pp. iii–iv, 7; Mynors, *Durham Cathedral Manuscripts*, p. 2, and nos. 91, 93, says there were originally seven volumes, of which two have survived. This is entirely likely, but, if the printed version edited by Botfield is correct, the catalog actually reports only four volumes for the first sixteen tracts. How the last ten were combined is not specified. See also Turner, "Earliest Durham Manuscripts"; Ker, *Medieval Libraries*, p. 255. The date is an inference from the fact that the listing of Herbert's books and those given by Prior Lawrence (1149–54) were in one twelfth-century hand and a list of books given by Prior Thomas (d. 1163) was added in another. The early dating is accepted by all scholars.

28. Cambridge University, Jesus College, Ms. Q D 2. For a description, see James, *Manuscripts in Jesus College*, p. 67, no. 44. I am grateful to D.J.V. Fisher for assisting me with this manuscript.

29. Edinburgh, The National Library of Scotland, Advocates Ms. 18. 6. 11. For a description, see *Summary Catalog of Advocates Manuscripts*, p. 111, no. 1442.

30. Sigerist, "Surgical Notebook," and "Early Medieval Medical Texts," esp. no. 3; Demaitre, "Theory and Practice in Medical Education," esp. p. 109.

31. A reference in Master Roger's book of surgery convincingly dates it to about 1170, but Herbert's copy must be an earlier version. Evidently 1170 denotes the year Master Guido of Aretino arranged and completed Roger's surgery, with the permission of the author, rather than the time it was first composed. Otherwise Herbert's pre-1153 collection and this particular work cannot be reconciled. For Roger see Corner, "Salernitan Surgery."

32. Dioscorides's *De Virtutibus Herbarum* is fos. 17–148 in the Jesus College Ms. For the herbal see Riddle, "Dioscorides." For the additions from the Saxon lapidary, see Kitson, "Lapidary traditions," pp 12, 57. Herbert of Durham's library once included a herbal by Macer Floridus, but it did not survive. The late eleventh-century work, probably compiled by Odo de Meung, near Loire, was a poorly arranged, sometimes medically dangerous, confused mass of material; Macer Floridus, esp. pp. 13–14; Flood, "Pliny and the 'Macer' Text."

33. For the text, identification with Philip, and sample facsimile of this lapidary (fos. 148–58 in the Jesus College Ms., see Meyer, "Les plus anciens lapidaires"; Studer and Evans, *Anglo-Norman Lapidaries*, pp. 265–76. See also Chapter 1, nn. 15 and 43.

34. Pedro's booklet is fos. 6–8v in the Jesus College Ms.

35. Mynors, *Durham Cathedral Manuscripts*, nos. 57 (Hunter Ms. 100, a particularly fine work of 1100x1128; see plates 37a, 37c); 71 (Glasgow University Library, Hunterian Ms. T, 4. 2, probably written shortly after 1140, as the death of Bishop Geoffrey Rufus is mentioned); 83 (Cambridge University, Sidney Sussex College, Ms. Δ 3.6).

36. Botfield, ed., *Catalog of Durham Cathedral*, p. 6. The library also possessed treatises on the astrolabe, the ecclesiastical calendar, and the abacus (p. 3), as well as the Bede's *De Tabernaculo*, all works used by other doctors. Herbert's copy of the Pantegri could have been recopied from the Cathedral library edition, Jesus College Ms. Q. B. 11; James, *Manuscripts in Jesus College*, p. 36, no. 28. Saint Augustine's Canterbury collected many of the same books Herbert had and used them frequently; Corpus Christi College, Cambridge, Ms. 466; James, *Manuscripts in Corpus Christi College*, 2:397. The earliest Salernitan works, however, may have come to England with the physician-abbot, Baldwin of Bury; Thomson, "The Library of Bury St. Edmund's," p. 634.

37. The 110 burgesses in Totnes in 1086 imply a population of 550. The 399 houses in Exeter in 1086 suggest 2,000 people; Darby and Finn, *Domesday Geography of South West England*, pp. 284, 281. Sometimes the estimated ratio of doctors received additional confirmation. When a Saxon named Ailsi, the father of two of Henry I's scribes, suffered great pain in his eyes he consulted several physicians before being healed by St. Stephen; see the account by his grandson, Peter of Cornwall, in Coulton, *Social Life in Britain*, pp. 221–26.

38. Salter, "City of Oxford," p. 98. In 1086 Warwick town had almost 250 houses and a population of 1,500; the borough had 6,896 people; Darby and Terett, *Domesday Geography of*

Midland England, p. 306. This is a higher town estimate than the 900 offered by H. A. Cronne, *The Borough of Warwick in the Middle Ages*, Dugdale Society, Occasional Papers no. 10 (Oxford: Oxford University Press, 1951), p. 12. York's population of about 9,000 in 1066 had declined to 4,000 or 5,000 by 1086; Darby and Maxwell, *Domesday Geography of Northern England*, pp. 154-56.

39. Barlow, ed., *Winton Domesday*, 1:440.

40. These figures are based on my analysis of Wickersheimer, *Dictionnaire Biographique*. Physicians in Normandy included: Abbot Gontard, who was at the Conqueror's deathbed; Giles of Saint Augustine, an important astrologer in the Conqueror's time; John of Rheims, who left William's court and entered the abbey of Saint Evroult; John of Arques, a famous astrologer and urologist at Rouen about 1125. Raoul, the ill-tonsured clerk who loved knightly sports, had studied at Salerno, where his only intellectual rival was a woman. He later became a monk at Marmoutier and Saint Evroult, successfully prayed to contract leprosy, and died in 1086. Both Goisbertus of Saint Evroult and Bishop Gilbert Maminot of Lisieux, a very avid astronomer, visited England. For continental practice, see Dubreuil-Chambardel, *Les Médecins* and MacKinney, *Early Medieval Medicine*. Wickersheimer made numerous correction of Dubreuil-Chambardel. Baudri, abbot of Bourgueil, dedicated a poem to the Conqueror's daughter, King Stephen's mother, Countess Adela of Blois, including a long description of contemporary medical practice and instruction; see Baudri of Bourgueil, pp. 196ff., lines 1254-1341; also in Dubreuil-Chambardel, pp. 54-56.

41. Orderic Vitalis, 1:89, 29; Wickersheimer, *Dictionnaire Biographique*, especially s.v. "Obizo," "Pierre Lombard," "Solomon," Jean de Dijon," "Thomas Falyn," and "Zour"; the last three were prominent astrologers.

42. Jadon, "Physicians of Syria," and "The Wealth, Prestige, and Medical Works of Physicians of Salah-al-Din." Only about eighty-five physicians are recorded with the Roman armies during their centuries of conquest; Majno, *The Healing Hand*, p. 390.

43. Some claimed he was more concerned with saving money than with improving his digestion; William of Malmesbury, *G.R.*, 2:483.

44. Talbot and Hammond, *Medical Practitioners*, p. 19.

45. Ibid, pp. 231-32.

46. *31 Henry I*, pp. 148-49.

47. Golb, "Forgotten Jewish History."

48. Roth, *History of the Jews*, p. 8.

49. Talbot and Hammond, *Medical Practitioners*, p. 199.

50. Thirty years after Wulfric's death, John of Ford composed his biography; John of Ford, *Wulfric of Haselbury*. Dennis Bethell is now preparing a new edition and translation.

51. Many of these observations have been persuasively argued by Mayr-Harting, "Functions of a Twelfth-Century Recluse," pp. 337-52.

52. John of Ford, *Wulfric of Haselbury*, p. 91.

53. Henry of Huntingdon, p. xxix.

54. Godric's sanctity impressed many people and was recorded by different monks of Durham — Germanus, Geoffrey, and Reginald — all of whom had some contact with the hermit; see Reginald of Durham, *Godric*. Reginald was also a great collector of miracles and had earlier compiled a study of Saint Cuthbert's healings.

55. Sumption, *Pilgrimage*, p. 123, 197. The bed count dates from about 1165.

56. Rotha Mary Clay, *The Hermits and Anchorites of England* (London, 1914), p. xxii.

CHAPTER III

1. William of Malmesbury, *G.P.*, pp. 194-95 and *G.R.*, 2:387-88. His earlier views can be detected in the parchment erasures. For John's career see Smith, "John of Tours"; Talbot and Hammond, *Medical Practitioner*, pp. 192-93; Barlow, *The English Church*, pp. 66-67, 263; Hunter, *Ecclesiastical Documents*; Gransden, *Historical Writing*, p. 181.

2. Barlow, *The English Church*, p. 263; Engels, "De obitu Willelmi," pp. 240-42.

3. Cunliffe, *Roman Bath Discovered*, pp. 1-2; *Regesta*, 1, nos. 314, 315, 326; *Regesta*, 2, no. 544 (a confirmation by King Henry in 1101). William's deed said the cost was 60 pounds, but William of Malmesbury (*G.P.*, p. 194) said it was 500 pounds.

4. *Gesta Stephani*, pp. 38–39; Henry of Huntingdon, p. 11.

5. William of Malmesbury, *G.P.*, p. 195. Among the few favors that John and his cathedral received were a general confirmation of privileges in 1101, a fair in 1102, and some more lands and rights in 1111; *Regesta*, 2, nos. 544, 573, 988, 989.

6. Henry of Huntingdon, p. 316. Of the twenty-six royal writs John attested, four were co-signed by Grimbald, the physician; *Regesta*, 2, nos. 544 (1101), 683 (1105), 684 (1105), 1245 (1120x1122). In 1106 John restored to his cathedral some of the things he had taken from it and donated others he had acquired by his own labors; Corpus Christi College, Cambridge, Ms. 111, fo. 113v.; *Bath Cartularies*, p. 51. As late as 1121 John was impartially presiding over involved disputes; Madox, *History of the Exchequer*, 1:109–12.

7. *Regesta*, 2, no. 1307, Latin text, p. 343, no. 144; Talbot and Hammond, *Medical Practitioners*, pp. 266–67; Patterson, *Gloucester Charters*, p. 146, no. 156. Interestingly, some of these lands later supported Picot, the physician. Late in the century a smith named Fulk appended to his charter the seal of Master Henry, the doctor of Nottingham, because he lacked a seal of his own; Holdsworth, *Rufford Charters*, 1:18.

8. *H.R.H.*, p. 121; Brooke and Keir, *London*, p. 321; *Regesta*, 2, nos. 734, 735, 1369, 1399.

9. Clarembald is mentioned five times:
—With Bishop Richard (1108–27) and Dean William of Saint Paul's (1108–38), as *medicus et capellanus*; printed twice by the *Historical Manuscripts Commission, Ninth Report*, pp. 31, 66;
—1115x1117 as medicus, attesting with Abbot Gilbert and William de Bocland; Robinson, *Gilbert Crispin*, pp. 154–55, a document that has generally escaped attention;
—About 1118 as medicus; witnessing a grant of Robert Fitz Martin to Totnes Priory; Watkin, *History of Totnes*, 1:26;
—1128x1131 as chaplain of the king, witnessing a grant of Bishop Warelwast to the new Launceston Priory; Lambeth Ms. 719, fo. 7v; cited by Rose-Troup, *Exeter Vignettes*, pp. 9–19; abridged in B.L. Ms., Lansdowne 939, fo. 21, cited by Oliver, *History of Exeter*, p. 21;
—About 1129, simply as Clarembald medicus, attesting a decision of Bishop Warelwast's court about Bernard, the scribe; Round, "Bernard," p. 421. See also Talbot and Hammond, *Medical Practitioners*, pp. 29–30.

10. For Master Odo see Luscomb, "Authorship of the *Ysagoge*." Luscomb apparently did not realize there was an Exeter canon named Master Odo. Gilbert Foliot, abbot of Glastonbury and bishop of London, evidently studied under Robert Pullen in Exeter. For more on Laon, see Chapter 4, n. 61.

11. For a valuable recent study, see Blake, "Bishop William Warelwast"; William of Malmesbury, *G.P.*, pp. 201–2.

12. *31 Henry I*, p. 157.

13. *Shrewsbury Cartulary*, 2:301, no. 329.

14. Bishop, *Liturgica Historica*, pp. 408–9, translated Hildebert's letter; see also Rose-Troup, *Exeter Vignettes*, pp. 15–16.

15. Osbert of Clare, pp. 110 (no. 31), 217–18. Williamson, the editor of Osbert's letters, suggested that Clarembald, the Cluniac prior of Bermondsey (1134–48) and abbot of Faversham (1148–77), could have been the recipient. Another candidate might be Clarembald, the prior of Montacute (1155–58), of Thetford (1158–63), and abbot of Saint Augustine's Canterbury (1163–73). His predecessor at Montacute was Prior Nicholas. See *H.R.H.*, pp. 36, 49, 114, 122, 125.

16. "Miracles of St. Cuthbert," p. 7. For Clarembald's property, see Oliver, *Monasticon Exoniensis*, p. 136.

17. This is Oxford University, Bodleian, Ms. 479, on whose flyleaf is written *Lib[er] Clerobaldi*; see Rose-Troup, *Exeter Vignettes*, pp. 9–19. Copies could be found at places like Salisbury, Winchester, Durham, Reading, Cirencester, and Rievaulx: Ker, "Salisbury Cathedral Library"; Botfield, ed., *Catalogues of Durham Cathedral*, p. 3; Barfield, "Lord Fingall's Cartulary" p. 120; Williams, "Gloucestershire Medieval Libraries," p. 76; James, *Manuscripts in Jesus College*, p. 48, no. 34.

18. Oliver, *Monasticon Exoniensis*, p. 136. Deeds of Bishop Warelwast and the Exeter chapter mention Clarembald's city property, which had formerly belonged to Ranulf de Haga. In neither charter was Clarembald called a physician.

19. Greenway, ed., *Le Neve's "Fasti,"* 1:61. For the other Nigels, see Appendix 1.

20. Ibid. Greenway once thought (p. 41) that Nigel, the nephew of Bishop Roger, who held Chiswick prebend, was Nigel of Calne. He was not, and Greenway's second volume deleted this identification; ibid., 2:111.

21. *Regesta*, 2, no. 1164; full text, *Register of Saint Osmund*, 1:239.

22. *Regesta*, 2, nos. 1204 (as chaplain, datable 1119 at Rouen); 1018 (1112, St. Mere Église); 1209 (1117x1119, Rouen); 1230 (1120, Caen, a gift to the Colchester infirmary); 1231 (1120, Caen).

23. *Winchester Cartulary*, p. 100. The editor dated this 1111x1114, but it must be earlier because the king confirmed the grant; *Regesta* 2, no. 884 (1102x1110). Another party to the agreement, Richard, became bishop of London only in 1108; hence the grant must be 1108x1110.

24. Kealey, *Roger of Salisbury*, p. 238; *31 Henry I*, p. 18

25. Everard's career is also confused by the coincidence that King Henry had two chaplains, Everard of Montgomery and Everard of Calne; see Landon, "Everard Bishop of Norwich"; Brett, *English Church*, pp. 108–10.

26. *31 Henry I*, p. 91. Oddly, the lands involved were in Norfolk. At the same time a certain Hugh of Monte Virum paid the exchequer two silver marks for the right to marry the mother of the bishop of Norwich (p. 54).

27. Richard of Calne is mentioned in 1130; ibid., pp. 23, 102, 126. An Everard of Calne attested a charter of the empress in 1144, but this must have been someone other than the bishop; *Regesta*, no. 111. Bishop Everard had a brother Arthur and at least ten nephews, including Adam, Peter, Richard, and William, who frequently attested his writs.

28. Most of the evidence for his life is found in the abbey cartulary, *Abingdon Chronicle*, esp. 2:44–158, 285–90. See also Talbot and Hammond, *Medical Practitioners*, pp. 45–46.

29. *Vita S. Aldelmi*, in *P.L.*, 89:63–84; the text is also in J. Bollandus and G. Henschenius, eds., *Acta Sanctorum Quotquot Toto Urbe Coluntur vel a Catholicis Scriptoribus Celebrantur*, 66 vols. (Antwerp: 1640–1770, Brussels: 1780–1925), 4:84 (25 May). The book was written after Abbot Warin's translation of Aldhelm's bones in 1080, which it mentions. Faritius knew and used Dominic of Evesham's "Life of St. Ecgwine"; see Dominic of Evesham, p. 73.

30. William of Malmesbury, *G.P.*, pp. 330–31; see also p. 126.

31. Ibid., pp. 192–93.

32. *Abingdon Chronicle*, 2:50.

33. Ibid., p. 55.

34. Ibid., pp. 44–55.

35. Ibid., p. 55; see also pp. 150–51, 286–89.

36. The monastery cartulary was edited by J. L. Fisher, (listed in bibliography under *Colne Cartulary*.)

37. P.R.O., Ms. E 132/2/13 m.1. I owe this reference to the kindness of Professor Robert B. Patterson of the University of South Carolina.

38. *Abingdon Chronicle*, 2:51–146.

39. Besides his friend Grimbald, Faritius also met Geoffrey and Rainier at Abingdon and no doubt remembered Gregory from Malmesbury.

40. Thirty–nine of Henry's writs mention Faritius by name, and although thirty–four others before 1118 were for his abbey, the abbot attested only three himself; *Regesta*, nos. 753, 825, 828.

41. *Abingdon Chronicle*, 2:289.

42. *P.L.*, 163:763–64. Theobald remarked that he was particulary fond of Abingdon's prior.

43. For relics, see *Abingdon Chronicle*, 2:42; for students, see 2:123, 137, 229, and Davis, "Henry of Blois."

44. *Abingdon Chronicle*, 2:287.

45. *Regesta*, 2, nos. 553, 576, 654, 697, 725, 789, 814, 815, 857, 952, 961, 974, 979, 983, 984, 1000.

46. Feudal aid, Ibid., no. 959, *Abingdon Chronicle*, 2:113; Domesday Book, *Regesta*, 2, no. 1000, *Abingdon Chronicle*, 2:115–16. (It was later called *Liber de Thesauro*); Writ of right, *Regesta*, 2, no. 974. Harvey "Domesday Book," p. 179, has recently expressed doubt that this treasury book was in fact Domesday.

47. *Regesta*, 2, no. 1000.

48. In 1114-15 Faritius acquired a house in Winchester, which he rented from the bishop of that city. Presumably the abbot wished a private place to stay when in town for government affairs. Many other ecclesiastics had such properties in London and Winchester; Barlow, ed., *Winton Domesday*, p. 389.

49. For a discussion of the election, see Kealey, *Roger of Salisbury*, pp. 125-28. The evidence is in the *Abingdon Chronicle*, 2:287; William of Malmesbury, *G.P.*, pp. 126-27; *Eadmer H.N.*, pp. 221-23.

50. Dubreuil-Chambardel, *Les Médecins*, pp. 184-85.

51. See Chapter 1, n. 53.

52. *Abingdon Chronicle*, 2:146-49.

53. Ibid., p. 290.

54. *Regesta*, 2, nos. 528a, 544, 567, 654, 683, 734 (spurious), 736, 758, 804, 812, 943. The Normandy attestations are nos. 1015, 1015a, 1017, 1439; also see Talbot and Hammond, *Medical Practitioners*, pp. 67-68. Grimbald's first attestation of a royal charter is confusing. A great concourse witnessed Henry's grant to the Cathedral of Bath in 1101, but the names are recorded somewhat differently in the two cartulary copies. Cambridge, Corpus Christi College, Ms. 111, fo. 103, a mid twelfth-century manuscript, reads Grimbald, the chaplain. This version was used by William Hunt in his edition of the *Bath Cartularies*, p. 43. B.L., Ms. Egerton 3316, fo. 87v, a fourteenth-century cartulary, reads Grimbald medicus. *Regesta*, 2, no. 544, follows this reading, although it does not report the later manuscripts in all other respects. According to a later description, Grimbald was clearly a husband and father, presumably in legal marriage. Perhaps the first version is a scribal error, corrected from a lost original by a later copyist.

55. *31 Henry I*, pp. 22, 46, 60, 76, 80; Barlow, ed., *Winton Domesday*, p. 127. In Leicester, Grimbald, almost certainly the physician, also held one-half a caracuate in Twyford from the king; Salde, *Leicestershire Survey*, pp. 15, 36, 84.

56. *Regesta*, 2, nos. 1369, 734; Colne Cartulary, p. 69, no. 31 (a grant of Aubrey de Ver).

57. *Regesta*, 3, no. 579 (November 1137 x January 1138 at Worcester).

58. He also held Thorne in Worcester from the bishop of Worcester; Cronne, "An Agreement Between Simon and Waleran."

59. John of Worcester, pp. 32-33.

60. William of Malmesbury, *G.R.*, 2:488.

61. Hollister, "Origins of the English Treasury," esp. pp. 267-68.

62. A late fourteenth- or early fifteenth-century example, probably made at Oxford, consisted of parchment pages folded 7 by 2 inches and contained drawings and treatises on astronomical prediction, bloodletting, and uroscopy; Talbot, "Vade Mecum."

63. The physician's name was Hugh, but he attested with the empress only in Rouen; *Regesta*, 3, nos. 88, 409, 432, 824. Gloucester's physician was Picot. Henry II has already been mentioned with Ralph and Robert de Veneys.

64. Facsimile, Andrews, "Charters of Reading Abbey"; cartulary copy, B.L. Ms. Egerton 3031, fo. 16. The original charter is still in private ownership.

65. *Oseney Cartulary*, 4:107. This is the only time he does not use the title *magister*, but the duplication of his fellow witnesses in other writs certifies that master and medicus Serlo are one and the same man.

66. —With Adeliza: (1) (1136) B.L. Ms. Egerton 3031, fo. 16v; (2) (1136x1139) original charter, New College Oxford, Stanton St. John charters, no. 26; facsimile, Salter, *Early Charters in Oxford*, no. 45; cartulary copy, *Eynsham Cartulary*, 2:172; (3) (1139x1140) original charter in B.L. Additional Charter 19573; facsimile, Kemp, *Reading Abbey*, p. 14; printed, Hurry, *Reading Abbey*, p. 158; cartulary copy, B.L., Ms. Harley 1708, fo. 20v; (4) (February 2, 1147) *Chichester Cartulary*, p. 23; (5) (1147x1150) Egerton 3031, fo. 16v. —With Earl William: (1) (1139x1140), Egerton 3031, fo. 43; Hurry, *Reading Abbey*, p. 159; (2) (c. 1148) Harley 1708, fo. 200v; Saltman, *Theobald*, p. 441; (3) (1142x1151) Egerton 3031, fo. 44v; (4) (c. 1160) B.L., Ms. Cotton Claudius A VI, fo. 37v; Dugdale, *Monasticon*, 4:645; *Boxgrove Cartulary* , p. 35. —With Jocelin: (1141x1151) Egerton 3031, fo. 37; printed, *E.Y.C.* 11:359, no. 289, —With Bishop Simon: (1125x1149) *Worcester Cartulary*, p. 39, no. 65.

Master Serlo also wrote to Bishop Simon about churches in Berkeley c. 1147, and Queen Adeliza attested the grant, Harley 1708, fo. 200v; Saltman, *Theobald*, p. 442, no. 218. Morey and Brooke, listed in bibliography under *Foliot Charters*, pp. 106–7, correctly suggest that identification of Serlo of Arundel with the poet Serlo of Wilton, is most unlikely. In the years immediately following 1147 the poet was on a Mediterranean island with many other English exiles; Friend, "Proverbs of Serlo of Wilton."

67. The evidence for this lengthy dispute is largely in Reading Abbey cartularies, especially B.L., Ms. Harley 1708, fo. 200v, which contains Serlo's writ, published in Saltman, *Theobald*, p. 442, no. 218, and in *Foliot Charters*, pp. 106–7, which contains Abbot Gilbert's letter. For the royal involvement, see *Regesta*, 3, nos. 695, 702, 706, 708, 709, 989. This whole quarrel has been sorted out by Kemp, in "Berkeley Hernesse." See also Sabin, "St. Augustine's Abbey and the Berkeley Churches"; ibid., Brooke, "St Peter of Gloucester," pp. 280–82.

68. The lands were at Aston, in Hertfordshire. The charter was the one that Master Serlo had witnessed as the clerk of the queen; see n. 64 above. Later, the monks forged a charter of King Stephen to "legalize" Adeliza's gift; *Regesta*, 3. no. 679.

69. Mayr-Harting, *"Acts of the Bishops of Chichester*, pp. 114–15, no. 55 (datable 1147x 1169, probably toward the early years); see also p. 10. A facsimile of Hilary's charter is reproduced as plate 5.

70. For bibliographies and brief accounts of Pedro's life, see Thorndike, *History of Magic*, 2:66–73; Haskins, *Medieval Science*, pp. 113–20; Sarton, *Introduction to the History of Science*, 2:199–201; O'Malley, "Petrus Alfonsi"; Hermes, ed., *"Disciplina Clericalis,"* pp. 3–99; Metlitzki, *Araby in Medieval England*, pp. 16–25, 95–106. The crucial research of the Spanish scholar José Maria Millás Vallicrosa is cited in succeeding notes. Pedro was not included in Talbot and Hammond, *Medieval Practitioners*. Lindberg, ed., *Science in the Middle Ages*, surveys the whole era in the light of the most recent research. The dating of Pedro's life and writing is complex and full of contradictions and I am trying to sort it out in greater detail in a study in progress, "Adelard of Bath, Pedro Alfonso, and Walcher of Malvern: A Scientific Triumvirate in Norman England."

71. For Pedro's godfather, see Lacarra, *Vida de Alfonso*, and Lourie, "Will of Alfonso I." For a valuable general history see O'Callaghan, *History of Medieval Spain*.

72. The full Latin text is in *P.L.*, 157:535–72. For a summary of its contents and context, see Williams, *Adversus Judaeos*, pp. 233–40. Some autobiographical parts were excerpted by Hermes, *"Disciplina Clericalis,"* pp. 35–40.

73. There are several editions of this work. I have used the one prepared by Eberhard Hermes and translated from the German by P. R. Quarrie. Another convenient English translation from the Latin is Joseph Ramon Jones and John Esten Keller, *The Scholar's Guide* (Toronto; Pontifical Institute of Medieval Studies, 1969). For an exhaustive literary analysis see Schwarzbaum, "Folklore Motifs in *Disciplina Clericalis.*" For some Hebraic influences on Pedro's tales, especially from the commentaries of Rashi of Troyes (1040–1105), see Metlitzki, *Araby in Medieval England*, pp. 102–3.

74. Corpus Christi College, Oxford University, Ms. 283, edited by Neugebauer, *Astronomical Tables of al-Khwarizimi* esp. pp. 134–35, 139, 181, 208, 218–19. For a discussion of the provenance of the manuscript, see Southern, *Medieval Humanism*, pp. 168–69. Surprisingly, these scholars did not mention each other's work.

75. Millás Vallicrosa, "La Aportación," pp. 87–97. There are several manuscript copies, such as Bodleian, Ms. Auct. F. 1. 9. fos. 96–99, from Worcester that included Walcher's earlier work and an edition of Adelard's al-Khwarizimi tables. Part of the *Dragon* was also published by Haskins, *Medieval Science*, pp. 116–17.

76. The longer version, B.L., Ms. Arundel 270, fos. 40v–45, was printed in Latin by Millás Vallicrosa in "La aportación," pp. 97–105. It was summarized by Thorndike, *History of Magic*, pp. 70–72, and translated by Hermes, *"Disciplina Clericalis,"* pp. 67–72, 75–80. Besides its rather free style, Hermes's translation is confusing in that it appears to treat two studies but in reality has only divided the *Letter on Study* into two parts. The shorter version, Corpus Christi College, Oxford University, Ms. 283, fos. 143v–145, is published in Latin and English by Neugebauer in *Astronomical Tables of al-Khwarizimi*, pp. 216–19. Part of the Latin text was also offered by Haskins, *Medieval Science*, pp. 117–18.

77. Cambridge University, Jesus College Ms. Q,D, 2. For more on this work, see Chapter 2, n. 28.

78. Hunt, "Disputation of Peter of Cornwall," p. 151.

79. Hermes, *"Disciplina Clericalis,"* p. 33. For the chronology, see Sarton, *Introduction to the History of Science*, 2:200, citing the work of M. Steinschneider.

80. The literature on Adelard is enormous, but for a perceptive, recent summary and bibliography, see Clagett, "Adelard of Bath." The case for connecting Pedro's and Adelard's work is most forcefully made by Millás Vallicrosa, *Nuevos estudios*, pp. 105-8; see also his "La Aportación," p. 82; Neugebauer, ed., *Astronomical Tables of al-Khwarizimi*, p. 230; Metlitzki, *Araby in Medieval England*, pp. 24-30, 47-55.

81. Southern, *Medieval Humanism*, pp. ix, 168-69, plates 7, 8. For John's handwriting see Ker, "Malmesbury Handwriting," p. 375. "The Chronicle of 'Florence'."

82. Thomson, "William of Malmesbury and Other Writers."

83. The entry on Henry I reads, "Dixit Petrus Amphulsus servus Jhesu Christi Henrici primi regis Anglorum medicus compositor huius libri"; from Cambridge University Library, Ms. Ii, vi, II, fo. 95 (a thirteenth-century manuscript of unknown origin). This was first noticed by Haskins, "Reception of Arabic Science," p. 60. Thorndike, *History of Magic*, 2:69, noted the odd usage of "the First."

84. Metlitzki, *Araby in Medieval England*, pp. 30-38, 60.

85. Lacarra, *Estudios de Edad Media*, 2:489-90, no. 20; 3:608. The first date was subsequently noticed by Millás Vallicrosa, "Un nuevo dato," p. 136; see also Hermes, ed., *"Disciplina Clericalis,"* p. 64.

CHAPTER IV

1. Clay, *Medieval Hospitals*, remains the only medieval survey on hospitals, but there is a very fine house-by-house summary by Knowles and Hadcock, *Medieval Religious Houses* (cited as *M.R.H.*). My tabulation differs slightly from theirs, and the documentation for additional or redated hospitals has been supplied in the list of Anglo-Norman hospitals in Appendix 2. The individual volumes of the *Victoria History of the Counties of England* (cited as *V.C.H.*) contain the best short descriptions of each institution. A very general account is given by Dainton, *England's Hospitals*.

2. Clay, *Medieval Hospitals*, pp. xviii, viii; Miller, "The Knights of Saint John." The dozens of early English hospitals specifically designated for the sick are not discussed by Miller. See also Woodings, "Medical Resources and Practice of the Crusader States." Many of the Crusader policies that Woodings mentions, such as fining physicians for poor treatment, had no parallel in England. If Eastern ideas were so important in Britain, one would have expected such practices to apply there, too.

3. Majno, *The Healing Hand*, pp. 382-83; Collingwood and Richmond, *Archaeology of Roman Britain*, pp. 15-69. The bath-hospital at Ravenglas, Cumberland, was founded by Edward Fitz Ulf, perhaps c. 1160x1180.

4. Bede, *Ecclesiastical History of the English People*, edited by Bertram Colgrave and Richard A. I. B. Mynors (Oxford: Oxford University Press, 1949). bk. 4, c. 31. This may have been a hospice. For Welsh place names see Cowley, *Monastic Order in South Wales*, p. 202.

5. See Chapter 2, n. 13.

6. These are: (1) Saint Wulstan, Worcester, 961x972; (2) Holy Trinity, Stow-on-the-Wold, Gloucester, 1010; (3) Saint Giles, Beverley, and (4) Saint Nicholas, Pontefract, the last two founded sometime before the Conquest.

7. Eadmer, *H.N.*, pp. 16-17.

8. A thirteenth-century cartulary remains, Cambridge University Library, Ms. Ll. 2. 15; *Saint Gregory's Cartulary*.

9. A Master Ebroin and a Master Lefwine attested Lanfranc's foundation charter. It is tempting to think that they were physicians, but they were probably schoolmasters; ibid., pp. 1-3: This charter is also published in Dickinson, *Origins of the Austin Canons*, pp. 280-82.

10. *Regesta*, 2, no. 1260 (1120x1133). William the almoner, chaplain, was a witness at Woodstock, and his presence suggests an early date, about 1121.

11. Gibson, *Lanfranc of Bec*, pp. 185-86.

12. Simanis, *National Health Systems*, p. 96; *New York Times*, Sunday, April 22, 1979.

13. See n. 50 for more on leprosy.

14. The story was repeated by William of Malmesbury, *G.R.*, 2:494; by Ailred of Rievaulx, see Clay, *Medieval Hospitals*, pp. 50-51; by annalist, *Aldgate Cartulary*, p. 223; by Matthew

Paris, *Chronica Majora*, 2:130; and by Roger of Wendover, *Flowers of History*, 1:459. For Matilda's reputation see Honeybourne, "Leper Houses, p. 5. See also *Dictionary of National Biography*, 13:52-53.

15. For Saint Giles see Honeybourne, "Leper Houses"; *V.C.H.*, *Middlesex*, 1:206-10; Parton, *St. Giles*. Brooke and Keir, in *London* (p. 319), observed that the foundation of Saint Giles, which was perhaps the earliest of the English leper hospitals, signified "an important epoch in medieval attitudes to social welfare." The praise would be better applied to Saint Nicholas Harbledown.

16. Brooke and Keir, *London*, pp. 32, 99, 315.

17. *Regesta*, 2, nos. 891, 926, 927.

18. Greenway, ed., *Charters of Mowbray*, pp. 6-14, 22-27, nos. 2-10, 23-31.

19. Ibid., p. 190, no. 287. Robert d'Aunay, Gundreda de Gournay, Roger de Mowbray, and the monks of Whitby also worked together to help found Byland Abbey at Hood, in the North Riding; ibid., p. 190, no. 288, pp. 27-57, n. 32-75.

20. Ibid., p. 196, no. 300 (1142x1154), p. 197, no. 302 (1154x1157); *M.R.H.*, p. 340.

21. *M.R.H.*, p. 402; *V.C.H.*, *Yorkshire*, 3:334.

22. *Regesta*, 2, nos. 1335, 1767.

23. *Regesta*, 2, nos. 1327 (1122, lands and privileges), 1328 (1122, wood for fuel and grass for cattle); 1889 (1123x1133, more land and general confirmation).

24. For Matilda's foundation see *V.C.H.*, *Sussex*, 2:80.

25. Matilda gave rents worth 20 pounds a year; *Regesta*, 3, no. 503 (1147x1152) and her husband's confirmation, no. 504 (1147–1152). The king did help set up Saint Giles's infirmary for the monks of Westminister; nos. 936–41 (1135–1154).

26. Ibid., 2, nos. 577 (1102), 1230 (1120).

27. *V.C.H.*, *Essex*, 2:185.

28. Barlow, ed., *Winton Domesday*, pp. x, 52, 328.

29. Harbledown: *Regesta*, 2, no. 1260 (1120x1133), ten perches of land around the hospital; Norwich: 1608 (c. 1129), 1855 (1123x1133), 1954 (1121x1133), tolls, tithes, and liveries of 3 pence a day—a good gift; Smithfield: 1761 (1133), 1794 (1133, a forgery), 1795 (1133), 1943 (1133x1135), valuable general liberties and churches; Chatham near Rochester: *V.C.H.*, Kent, 2:216, a penny a day for each patient.

30. Derby 74 pence; *31 Henry I*, p. 12. Perhaps this was for Saint Leonard's leper hospital, known to exist before 1171. The other Derby foundations seem slightly later—Saint Helen (c. 1146) and Saint James (c. 1140). For other general alms in 1129–30, see pp. 24, 44, 76, 109, 126, 131, 135, 137, 141. Additional charities are hidden under pardons and payments to various churches.

31. For example, at Colchester; *Regesta*, 2, nos. 577 (1102), 1230 (1120).

32. —The leper house at Pont-Audemer: *Regesta*, 2, no. 1918 (1135, a fair); 3, no. 663 (1135x1154). King Stephen's writ claims that Henry founded the establishment and persuaded Waleran of Meulan to build it. The viceroy also aided this house; Kealey, *Roger of Salisbury*, pp. 256-57 (the charter may be later, but the gift was Roger's). —The hospital at Falaise: *Regesta*, 2, nos. 1742 (1133, a mill and general confirmation), 1764 (1133, general confirmation), —The leper hospital at Rouen: *Regesta*, 3, no. 730 a very large gift of forty shillings a month, confirmed by Geoffrey of Anjou (1144-50); —the sick at Boulogne: *Regesta*, 2, no. 1924 (1125–1135), confirmation of a gift of Count Eustace repeated by Stephen as count. —For Chartres: *Regesta*, 2, no. 1917 (1135) a gift of ten pounds a year. This was slightly altered by his successors; *Regesta*, 3, nos. 69, 70, 71, 72.

For more, see Chapter 5.

33. Clay, *Medieval Hospitals*, p. 170. Unfortunately, I have not been able to find the original grant creating this fund.

34. York: *Regesta*, 3, nos. 989 (1135x1139, a grant of protection); 990 (1136x1139, freedom from gelds and a confirmation); 991 (1140, freedom from lawsuits); 992 (1146, forest grant); 993 (1154, forty shillings a year); 994 (1148x1154, mills and tolls). Colchester: 240 (1136x1152, fourteen acres worth 63d a year). General confirmations: to Saint Paul's Norwich, 619 (1135x 1140); Saint Bartholomew's, Oxford 636 (1136x1139); Partney Hospital, Lincoln 652 (1135x 1140); Pont-Audemer 663 (1135x1154), 749 (1137); Falaise 298 (1137), see also 299 (1150x 1151, Duke Henry's confirmation); Chartres: 69 (1137), 70 (1140), 71 (1150x1151, a charter of the empress and young Henry); 72 (1151x1153, empress and young Henry). Stephen did grant

lands and issue what seems to have been a foundation charter to the nuns of the hospital of Saint Mary and Saint John in Norwich; 615 (1136x1137). In 1146 two nuns of the hospital founded nearby Carrow Priory; *H.R.H.*, p. 216.

35. *Registrum Antiquissimum*, 3, no. 920 (1123x1135); Dyson, "Bishop Alexander," pp. 12–13; B.L., Harley Charter 45 C 32 (a grant of Adam of Amundeville to Elsham). *M.R.H.* (p. 351) dates the Carlton hospital after 1180, but Elias died before 1179. Also see Owen, *Church and Society*, p. 51.

36. *V.C.H.*, *Buckinghamshire*, 1:392.

37. Saltman, *Theobald*, pp. 279, 305, 411; see also pp. 386, 534, 539.

38. Thomas of Monmouth, *Saint William of Norwich*, p. 31.

39. For a particulary early set of customs, see Chapter 5.

40. Clay, *Medieval Hospitals*, p. 150.

41. Much of the evidence for Robert's career is in the different volumes of *E.Y.C.*

42. This establishment is unusually well documented: Moore, *History of St. Bartholomew's*, and *Book of the Foundation of St. Bartholomew's*; Webb, ed. *Records of St. Bartholomew's*, and *Book of the Foundation of the Church*; Kerling, "Foundation of St. Bartholomew's"; *St. Bartholomew's Cartulary*; Medvei and Thornton, eds., *Royal Hospital*.

43. Kealey, *Roger of Salisbury*, p. 76; Webb, ed. *Records of St. Bartholomew's*, 1:39–42. The decision to separate the hospital and priory was apparently made before 1133, but a new incumbent had not yet been chosen. One of Henry's writs refers to Rahere, the prior of the church, and to an unnamed prior of the hospital; *Regesta*, 2, no. 1761 (before 1133). Another royal grant was made about the same time, but was not included in the *Regesta*, Moore, *History of St. Bartholomew's*, 1:39–42.

44. Moore, *History of St. Bartholomew's*, p. 21; Webb, ed. *Records of St. Bartholomew's*, A writ of Earl David, Queen Matilda's brother, about property in Tottenham, London, was attested between 1114 and 1124 by Aelfric, a priest of Saint Bartholomew's; Lawrie, ed., *Early Scottish Charters*, p. 48.

45. *Regesta*, 2, nos. 1761 (1133), 1943 (1133x1135); see also 1794 and 1795 (forgeries).

46. Webb, ed. *Book of the Foundation of the Church*, pp. 18–19.

47. Ibid.; Medvei and Thornton, *Royal Hospital*, p. 104.

48. Webb, ed. *Book of the Foundation of the Church*, p. 25.

49. Ibid., p. 49.

50. Wells, "Leper Cemetery"; at Rubin, *Medieval English Medicine*, pp. 159, 166. See also MacArthur, "Medieval Leprosy"; Richards, *Medieval Leper; Mercier, Leper Hospitals*. A stimulating discussion of leprosy on the continent can be found in Simone C. Mesmin's unpublished 1978 Ph.D. thesis from the University of Reading, "The Leper Hospital of Saint Giles de Pont-Audemer: An Edition of its Cartulary and an Examination of the Problem of Leprosy in the Twelfth and Early Thirteenth Century."

51. Wells, *Bones, Bodies, and Disease*, p. 102.

52. Ibid., p. 94.

53. B.L., Ms. Egerton 3031 (Reading Cartulary), fo. 11v.

54. From the regulations of Abbot Thomas of Saint Albans (1349–96) for the leper hospital of Saint Julian; *Saint Alban's Chronicle*, 4(2):503.

55. *V.C.H.*, *Northamptonshire*, 2:162; King, *Peterborough Abbey*, pp. 27–28, 38.

56. Knowles, *Monastic Order*, pp. 136–37.

57. Thompson and Grace Goldin, *The Hospital*, offer a general analysis of building design, but there is not much on early England.

CHAPTER V

1. Jack, "An Archival Case History"; Roberts, "Llanthony Priory."

2. The *Registrum Magnum* is P.R.O., Ms. C 115/K 2/6683 (formerly called C 115/A 1). I am very grateful to Professor Christopher R. Cheney of Corpus Christi College, Cambridge University, for leading me to this document and helping me with its complications.

3. The original Latin text reads as follows.

   Hec est regula infirmorum de Dudeston edita ab Yvone magnifico Carnotensi episcopo summe discrecionis viro.

Ante omnia et super omnia ab infirmis observanda est obediencia paciencia castitas pro-
prieta[ti]s nuditas. Sint autem divisi viri a mulieribus nec viri ingrediantur domum femi-
narum nec femine vivorum sine licencia magistri. Captiulum festis diebus infirmis post sex-
tam teneatur, ubi de disciplinis suis corrigantur. Dominica + feria III^a et feria V^a si fieri
potest carnes accipiant. Ceteris autem diebus nisi festivitas observabilis supervenerit absti-
neant. Si quis autem de insufficienti oblacione ciborum vel potum murmuraverit, usque
tercio corripiatur. Si vero postea fecerit murmur servisie pocio usque satisfaccionem ei
tollatur, quia filii I[s]rael, propter murmuracionem in deserto mortui sunt. Preter duos vesti-
menta fratrum et sororum sique sint, unius sint coloris et non varii, silicet nigri, albi, vel
russeti. Suscepti autem fratres aut sorores promittant stabilitatem in loco et obedienciam
magistro qui preest. Infirmi non exeant foras soli, nec circumeant vicos set cum famulo vel
socio eant ordinati ubi imperatum fuerit. Infirmi post completorium non loquantur, nisi hii
qui in lecto omnino decumbunt. In ecclesia non loquantur, nisi in capitulo dum negocia
tractabunt. Siquis autem clamatus fuerit, prostratus veniam petat et humiliter confiteatur si
fecit id de quo clamatus est, vel neget si non fecit. Magistri autem qui secundum modum
discipline que iniungat ei penitenciam virgarum vel ieiuniorum. Siquis autem renuerit ac-
cipere disciplinam, sicut est ordo Cisternensis de communi societate expellatur. Siquis autem
in manifestam fornicacionem inciderit, absque ulla misercordia de societate expellatur. Siquis autem cum magistro contenciosus fuerit, acrius corripiatur, si ex consuetudine hoc
fecerit, proiciatur. Hospites infirmi adventantes caritative recipiantur, qui una nocte secundum facultatem domus serviantur. Ad horam divini officii summo mane surgant, et matu-
tinas de die et de Sancti Maria audiant. Laici autem pro matutinis dicant XXIIII pater noster.
Pro unaquaque hora dicant quinquies pater noster, pro vesperis sepcies, pro completorio
quinquies. Bis in die commedant omni tempore nisi in principalibus ieiuniis, set hora
debita. Omnes debent scire pater noster et ave Maria et Credo. Siquis autem sanus se reddi-
derit ad serviendum infirmis, promittat obedienciam et castitatem et vivat sicut constiterit ei
custos infirmorum. Nullus in mensa loquatur, nisi de necessariis, nec post completorium ali-
quis loqui presumat, nisi de necessariis domus tractandis. Nullus in civitatem vel villam
pergat nisi per licenciam magistri, et bene inquirat de illo negocio pro quo iturus est. Et si
vadat ante prandium veniat ad prandium; et si vadat post prandium veniat ad vesperas. Qui
istud mandatum non servaverit, caritatem XX dierum amittat.^{a} Nullus fratrum inveniatur
cum aliqua sorore vel soror cum fratre, in cellario vel in lardario vel in virgulto vel in orto
super caritate XL dierum.^{b} Explicit ista regula infirmorum, edita ab Yvone magnifico Carnotensi episcopo.

---

^{a}I cannot quite translate this as it stands and suspect there is a copyist error here. Literally it
seems to mean "(Let there be) masters who (act) according to the custom of the disciplne that
imposes on him a penance of rods and fasting."
^{b}A *caritas* is a technical monastic term for a special allowance of food or drink. I have rendered
these sentences somewhat freely on the basis that the punishment consisted in a loss of these
treats.
  I am indebted to the Reverend William H. Fitzgerald, S.J., of the College of the Holy Cross
for help in translating this text, and to Professor Bennett Hill of the University of Illinois and
the Reverend M. Basil Pennington, O.C.S.O., of Saint Joseph's Abbey, Spencer, Massachusetts, for additional commentary.
  4. Rose Graham, in *V.C.H.* (*Gloucester*, 2:121); believed that it was founded soon after
1150 and that it was intended for women; Knowles and Hadcock, in *M.R.H.* (p. 360), followed
her interpretation.
  5. Only Walter's general confirmation of all his gifts to Llanthony still exists; *Registrum
Magnum*, fo. 64. This was ratified by King Henry in 1125x1127, ibid. (not calendared in
Regesta, 2). Miles's charter did not specifically mention the hospital either, but a confirmation
by Bishop Simon of Worcester (1125–50) noted that half of Barrington had been given to the
poor of Dudston. This was also affirmed by Bishop Robert of Hereford (1131–48), who reported
that the grant was made in King Henry's time; *Registrum Magnum*, fos. 64v–65, for all three

writs. Earl Roger's grant, ibid., fo. 64, was published by David Walker, *Charters of Hereford*, pp. 24–25, no. 27. The Empress Matilda also gave, or confirmed, Barrington lands to Llanthony, some of which formerly had belonged to William of Buckland; *Registrum Magnum*, fo. 64; published in *Regesta*, 3, no. 497 (1141). William's own charter is also on fo. 64.

6. *Registrum Magnum*, fo. 64v.

7. Pipe Rolls, *2 Henry II*, p. 49; *3 Henry II*, p. 100; *4 Henry II*, p. 167. Thereafter, the grant continued to be made annually.

8. In 1159x1169 a Maurice of Hereford attested at Dudston (the place, not necessarily the hospital); Walker, *Charters of Hereford*, p. 45, no. 72. This may be the same man as Master Maurice, medicus, who witnessed with Bishop Robert Foliot of Hereford in 1174x1186; P.R.O., Ms. C 115/K 6679 (formerly C 115/A 9), fos. 126–126v, another Llanthony cartulary.

9. Le Grand, *Statuts d'hôtels-dieu*, pp. 7–11, 181–83.

10. I came upon the text of the Reading regulations too late to include them in this study, but I hope to edit them at another time. There are at least two copies, B.L., Ms. Egerton 3031, fo. 11v and B.L., Ms. Cotton Vespasian EV, fos 38–39. These rules could easily predate those at Jerusalem and Montpellier. A detailed set of later twelfth-century customs includes many provisions for care of the sick at a monastic infirmary; Clark, *Observances at St. Giles*, especially chaps. 45–46. Proper hospitals probably functioned in much the same way. The text seems to assume that the physician who visits the sick would be a layman. Naturally, there is much discussion about bleeding.

11. Stevenson, "A Calendar of the Records," pp. 426–27.

12. Dereene, "Les Coutumes de Saint Quentin," p. 411–12. For Ivo's advice to a convent of nuns, see Cambridge University, Corpus Christi College, Ms. 308, fos. 108–12; James, *Manuscripts in Corpus Christi College*, 2:108–9. For Ivo's life, see R. Spranel, *Ivo von Chartres* (Stuttgart, 1962.)

13. Ivo of Chartres, p. 469.

14. *Regesta*, 2, no. 1917 (1135). This grant was slightly altered by his successors; *Regesta*, 3, nos. 69–72. The original subsidy probably began between 1121 and 1131, but the surviving charter was reissued after the first had been burned. For the commercial exemption see *Beaulieu Cartulary*, p. 2, no. 2 (omitted from *Regesta*, 2). Waleran of Meulan was also a benefactor, *Beaulieu Cartulary*, p. 14, no. 29.

15. Le Grand, *Statuts d'hôtels-dieu*, pp. 214–23.

16. New information about Pont-Audemer appears in Mesmin, "The Leper Hospital of Saint Giles de Pont-Audemer." For this grant, see 1:79, 87. For Henry's initiative and Stephen's testimony, see *Regesta*, 3, no. 663 (1135x1150). For the bishop's role, see Kealey, *Roger of Salisbury*, pp. 256–57. Mesmin persuasively argued (1:240–60) that a charter I had attributed to Bishop Roger for Pont-Audemer must belong to a later Bishop R. of Salisbury, but there is no question that the original tithes of Sturminster Dorset came from Roger.

17. Clerval, *Les Écoles des Chartres*, p. 180.

18. His life was recorded by a Llanthony canon, William of Wycumbe, who later became fourth prior of the monastery; Henry Wharton, *Anglia Sacra Sive Collectio Historiarum de Archiepiscopis et episcopis Angliae ad Annum 1540*, 2 vols. (London, 1691), 2:293–300. For attestations of a Robert de Bethune with Robert Count of Flanders, see *Regesta*, 2, nos. 515 (1101), 941 (1110).

19. The Cistercian Constitutions were mentioned in the undated foundation charter of Pontigny Abbey, probably written in 1114, and in a bull of Pope Calixtus II in 1119. Stephen Harding's predecessor, Abbot Alberic (1099–1109), may have also drawn up statutes; Lekai, *The Cistercians*, pp. 18–32, 442–66.

20. It is remotely possible that the Llanthony copyist confused Bishop Ivo with another author. An Englishman named Ivo was one of the first Cistercians at Clairvaux; Knowles, *Monastic Order*, p. 228. A Master Ivo of Chartres taught theology at Chartres about 1179; Smalley, "Master Ivo of Chartres", Baldwin, *Masters, Princes, and Merchants*, 1:315, 332. The bishop however is certainly the preferred author, however.

CHAPTER VI

1. Henry of Huntingdon, pp. 254–58.

2. Kealey, "King Stephen," and "Anglo-Norman England."

INDEX

Since surnames were still relatively rare in the early twelfth century, all medieval persons in this index are listed by their given names. The terms *Fitz* and *son of* are almost interchangeable, but the title *master* is usually not included for physicians. Abbreviations used are: abb. = abbot; abp. = archbishop; bp. = bishop; pr. = prior. Physicians listed only in Appendix 1 are not included here.

Edward J. Kealey is professor of history at the College
of the Holy Cross in Worcester, Mass. He is the author of
Roger of Salisbury, Viceroy of England.

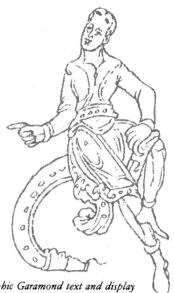

The Johns Hopkins University Press
This book was composed in Compugraphic Garamond text and display
type by Britton Composition Company from a design by Susan
Bishop. It was printed on 50-lb. number 66 Eggshell Offset cream
paper by Universal Lithographers, Inc., and bound in Joanna Arrestox
cloth by The Maple Press Company.